Herbal Medicine for Emotional Healing

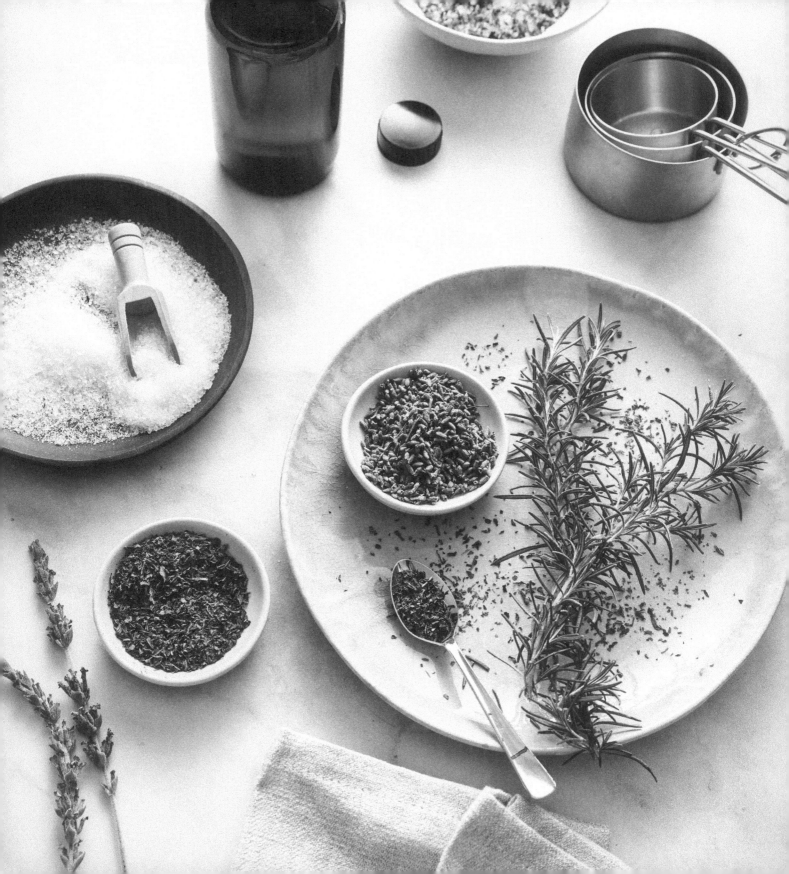

Herbal Medicine
for Emotional Healing

101 NATURAL REMEDIES FOR ANXIETY, DEPRESSION, SLEEP, AND MORE

Tina Sams

Photography by Alicia Cho

ROCKRIDGE
PRESS

Interior and Cover Designer: Angie Chiu

Art Producer: Karen Williams

Editor: Clara Song Lee

Production Editor: Nora Milman

Photography © Alicia Cho, styling by Ashley Nevarez, pp. ii, vi, xii, xvi, 2, 10, 20, 28, 30, 52, 66, 76, 84, 106, 142; © Helene Dujardin pp. 109, 113, 114, 115, 118, 121, 122, 124, 129, 135, 136, 139; © Lucia Loiso pp. 132, 126; shutterstock pp. 108, 111, 112, 117, 133, 138; istock pp. 116, 119, 120, 123, 125, 127, 130, 131, 140.

Author photo © Lori Stahl.

ISBN: Print 978-1-64611-997-4 | eBook 978-1-64611-998-1

R0

TO MY MAIN PARTNER IN ADVENTURES
AND LAUGHTER, MY SISTER MARYANNE,
WHO STARTED US ON THIS HERBAL JOURNEY.

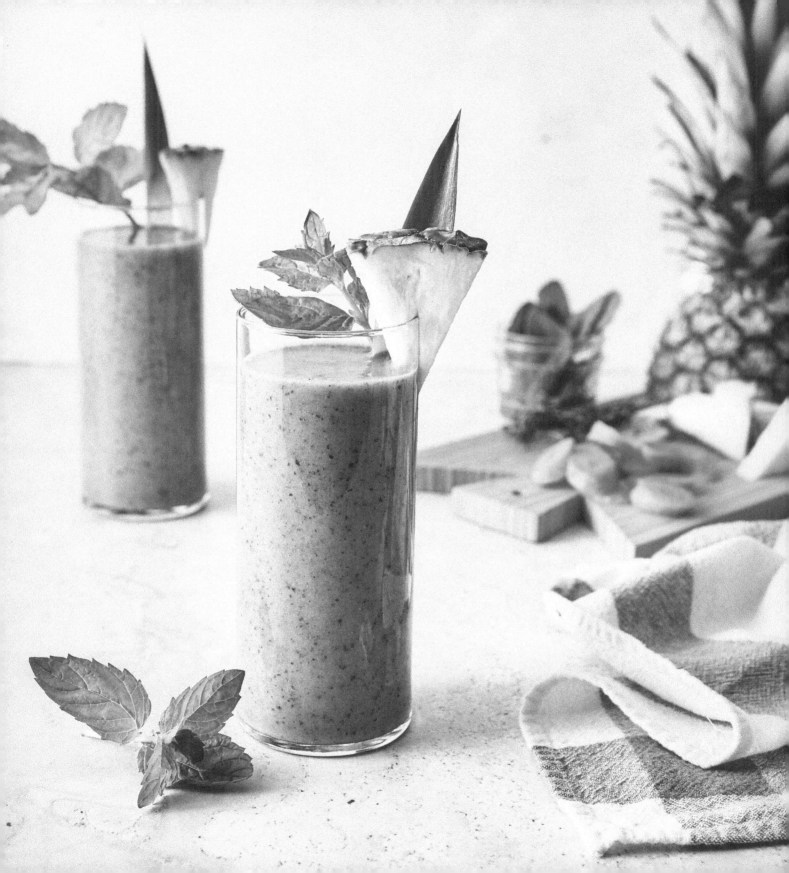

Contents

Part Three: Herbal Allies for Emotional Work

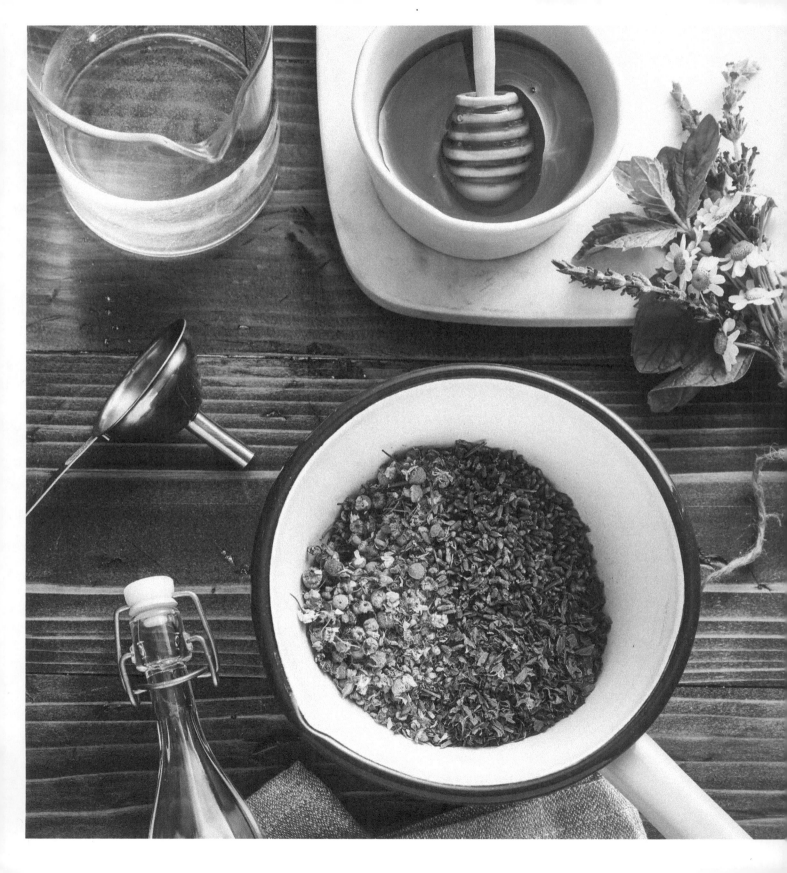

Introduction

Welcome to what may be a new way of approaching wellness for you. Most people have used herbal medicine in one way or another, even if that was simply taking orange juice to discourage a cold or wild cherry lozenges to quell a cough. It may be a novel idea for you to turn to herbs for your emotional health. I'm here to show you how these gentle yet effective plant medicines can provide profound support during difficult times, whether that looks like low-lying depression, an acute anxiety attack, insomnia, stress-related pain, or any other affliction that keeps you from shining your light and feeling the full extent of your vitality.

In *The Essential Herbal*, Toronto-based herbalist Cathy Walker perfectly describes the ineffable power of herbs to help people heal:

> I wasn't just giving them tea, I was giving them all the beauty that surrounded each plant. I was filling their emptiness with the swamps, the meadows, and every plant's experiences of deer running past them, rabbits feasting on them, sound of trains off in the distance. Thunderstorms and brilliant sunrises, breathtaking sunsets and long winter nights with full moons shining down on them all, along bubbling creeks and streams, rushing rivers and huge waves from gigantic lakes, the quietness of the forest, and all the colours that changed with each season. I knew when they drank [the tea], they were drinking in all of those experiences that each of the plants had to share and that would heal them far deeper than I ever could.

I love this description because when I tell someone that learning about a few healing herbs will empower them, it doesn't quite encompass the intensity of the experience. Cathy better illustrates how deeply plants can soothe one's soul as well

as how integrated we all are: humans, plants, the planet—and even the universe. It is very powerful.

We have always been surrounded by plants. They feed you, provide you with shelter, and can be woven into cloth. They can also heal you. Take a moment to look around right now. You will probably see décor nearby that has some type of plant, flower, or leaf motif. If you're wearing a fragrance, it is most likely made from either plants or a chemical blend that mimics plants. All creatures need plants. They've been on Earth much longer than we have, and some folks feel that the herbs care for us and want us to be well. I agree. When your emotional or spiritual health feels fragile, herbs are your strong allies.

Some regard herbs as only the seed-bearing plants that have nonwoody stems and die down to the ground every year, while others say they are *any* plant with seeds, leaves, and flowers. I go one step further and apply a much broader interpretation that includes any plant, tree, root, fruit, seed—and

some mushrooms. The world of herbs has expanded exponentially in the past few decades, and we all benefit from that.

In my part of the country, you can't walk 10 feet without finding a wild plant that will soothe your mind, body, or spirit. Visiting friends in Manhattan, I was pleasantly surprised to find that birds had seeded their rooftop garden with some wonderful healing "weeds." Generally speaking, herbs work gently with few side effects. They're everywhere! Knowing just a few herbs allows you to take your wellness into your own hands. By turning to herbs to calm your mind and settle—or spark—your spirit, you will embark on an empowering, never-ending adventure. I hope that's where this book leads you.

It's important to realize that herbs work because they have strong components and actions. Even though they are usually gentler than drugs and might take a while to work, they need to be respected. In fact, most pharmaceutical drugs include synthetically made herbal constituents. Just because something

is natural does not necessarily mean that it is safe. The sun-loving desert plant ephedra (*Ephedra sinica*) is a good example: While extremely effective for respiratory issues, particularly asthma, it is also a stimulant. Thinking that it was natural so it was safe, it was concentrated (not by herbalists, I might add) to make "herbal speed," sold everywhere, and people died. Now it is illegal in the United States and unavailable to all of us.

In addition, the idea that herbs and allopathic medicine don't go together is a myth. Doctors are not our enemies. To begin with, a good diagnosis is critical in any kind of chronic condition, and emotional issues that don't improve—or worsen—should be addressed by a mental health professional or family physician. Nobody would suggest an herb for a heart attack, so when something is severely impacting your mental or emotional health to the point that daily life is challenging, it deserves to be treated just as seriously and with the same care and understanding. If you are under treatment for a chronic condition or take medication regularly, please check with your doctor before starting to use herbs.

In the following pages, you'll find lots of supportive herbal allies, and you'll learn how to best prepare them so you can start to feel better. There is a medicine maker's guide that simply walks you through how to create the herbal preparations that are most effective for strengthening emotional well-being. You'll find 101 tried-and-true recipes and remedies for more than 30 conditions that are related to anxiety, depression, stress, grief, and more. I also share profiles for 31 of my favorite herbs for emotional healing and well-being. Let's get started.

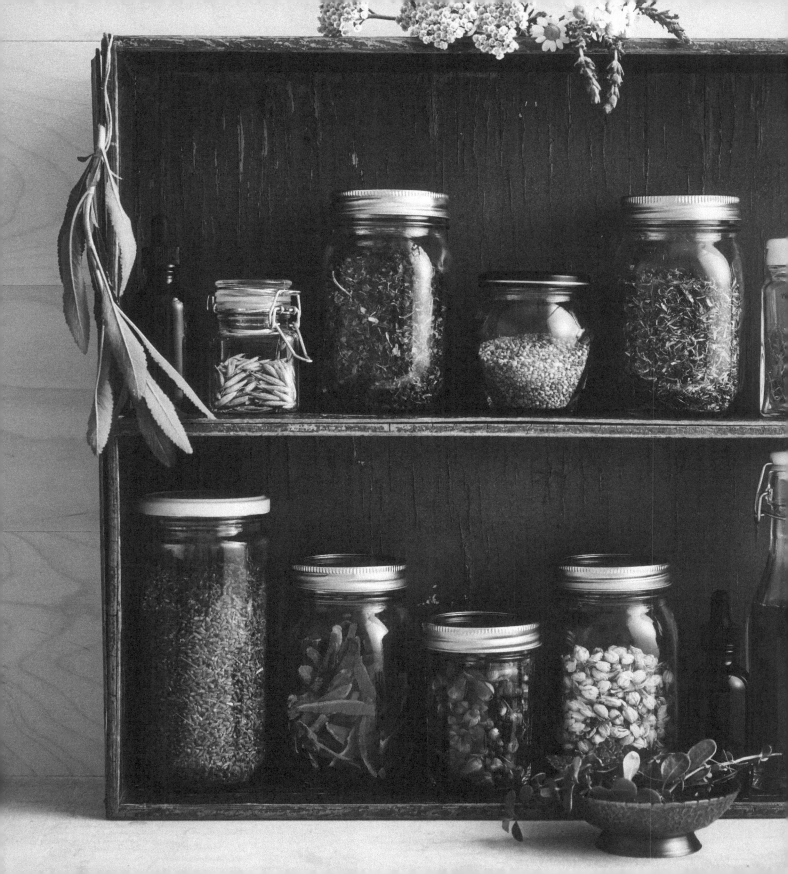

PART ONE

The Medicine Maker's Guide

Herbs have been used for medicine and comfort for all of recorded history with written records going back as far back as 1500 BCE. Less than 100 years ago, herbs were the only medicines we had, and they can still be used today to bring about health, well-being, and spiritual experiences through ceremony. When you open up to them, you'll find yourself much happier from spending a mere 30 minutes out in the woods or the meadow, communing with the plants.

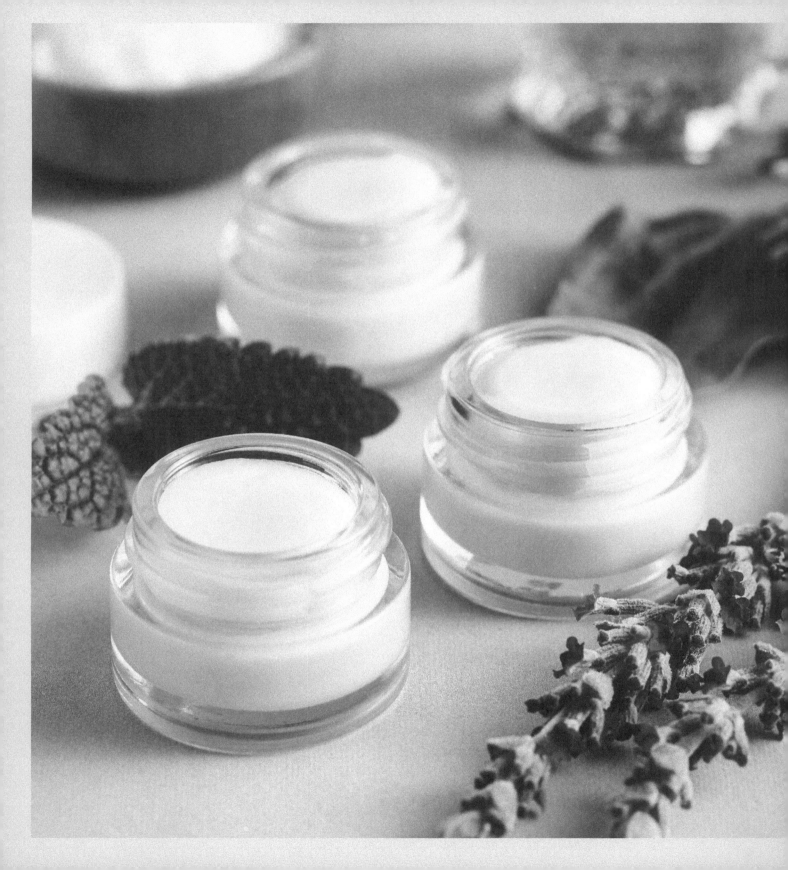

CHAPTER 1

How Herbal Medicine Heals

There are many different emotional states, most of which are a normal and healthy part of life. Emotional states that are considered "positive," such as happiness, relaxation, and contentment, often improve your health, whether by releasing endorphins that trigger pleasurable feelings or by calming your body's immune system and stress responses. Emotional states that are considered "negative," such as fear, stress, and sadness, can feel less pleasant but under normal circumstances may also be helpful, since they can protect you from danger or alert you to problems that need addressing.

When emotional states become overwhelming or chronic, or disrupt your life too much, issues can arise. While herbal medicine can't *always* fix emotional problems, it can often ease them. Physical manifestations of emotions—whether due to heartbreak, stress, depression, abandonment, loneliness, anxiety, or other emotional disruptors—can often be improved with herbs, too. In this chapter, we'll learn about how herbal medicine can help us manage challenging emotional states.

A Holistic Approach to Health

When you first start learning about herbs, you'll likely want to focus on their uses. A plant may provide scores of benefits, and learning that an herb will help you sleep better is great, but's what causing your insomnia in the first place? Herbalists like to take a holistic approach. It's important for a lot of reasons. For example, some herbs raise blood pressure, thin the blood, or interfere with the effectiveness of lifesaving medications. We have to be aware of all the actions of the herbs and all the needs of the individual before formulating a treatment.

Herbs are packed with vitamins, minerals, and trace elements. Many of the herbs we use as seasonings are healing powerhouses. When you start looking into herbs, you'll realize that there is a recurring theme: They'll protect us if we let them. The strongly scented herbs contain large amounts of essential oils, and all have antibiotic and antibacterial properties. Likewise, there are diuretic herbs, herbs that help wounds heal, and herbs that lessen pain. There's a huge array of helpers in the garden just waiting to be discovered! Herbs also contain built-in buffers. Sometimes, industry will come along and decide to extract just one component from an herb, turning it into something very similar to a drug. I always advocate using whole herbs, as their many constituents are designed to work synergistically.

The stronger and healthier our bodies are, the easier it is to address any kind of imbalance that comes along, whether it's physical, emotional, or spiritual. We have reserves of energy and feel resilient when we're healthy, but when our bodies are struggling to get into balance, that energy gets used up, making it easier for any illness to gain a foothold. Herbs, good food, good sleep, and exercise in fresh air can all help us stay healthy.

Herbalism for Emotional Healing

Herbal medicine is uniquely suited to assist us with our emotional, mental, and spiritual health. Many people (including myself) believe plants want to help us. Plants were on Earth long before humans and have much to share with us. For example, humans have an endocannabinoid system, with receptors throughout the brain and body, and research is showing how pain, disease, and the mind are all wired for cannabis. How many other plants will we discover that we are made to interact with?

Additionally, it's been found that there are microbes in soil that make us happy! Playing in the dirt causes a process that releases serotonin. Walk barefoot on the ground. It's good for you. In fact, there is a practice known as "grounding" or "earthing" that has been shown to affect us in many ways, such as reducing pain and improving sleep.

Herbs have so many benefits, not the least of which is helping us move toward balance. If you are stressed beyond belief, have trouble focusing, can't stay awake, or are completely leveled by grief, herbs are here to help. There are scores of herbs for each of these issues, and adversely, there are a couple that would help with every single one of them. Herbs really are that miraculous. Personally, I have found that rose, chamomile, and holy basil (among others) could each be used alone or in a combination for feelings ranging from a racing mind to deep sadness.

External physical conditions can arise from emotional imbalances. Stress can bring on an incredible number of symptoms that run the gamut from acne to life-threatening autoimmune diseases. You struggle on, telling yourself, "It's just stress," but you need to stop doing that. Depression linked to life events affects your body just like stress. Almost anytime you experience a negative life event, your body responds physically. Your immune system is usually compromised, and that starts the ball rolling. By finding and addressing the root cause of the emotional upset first, you can usually find ways to help with herbs. For serious problems, I urge you to find a clinical herbalist or homeopath or consult your primary care physician. You're worth it.

Herbs are empowering. Making your own medicine is exhilarating. Growing or gathering your own medicine is exciting. Learning about herbal remedies is amazing. Besides the fact that they are affordable compared to pharmaceuticals, every time you take control of your own care, you take a step toward strengthening your emotional well-being.

How Herbal Energetics Work

Herbal "energetics" is a term that refers to the fact that herbs, people, and symptoms all have defining characteristics, and we try to match herbs with people in ways that correct imbalances in energy (which manifest as symptoms of illness). The properties most used are hot/cold, dry/moist, and tense/lax. The easiest examples to me are the dry/moist energetics because I think we see them the most often. For a dry, hacking cough, a nice moistening tea or lozenge is most soothing. We may want a cooling herb to calm that hot, dry throat and a relaxing herb for the tension in the chest and shoulders. Seems pretty simple, right? I think a lot of it becomes second nature once herbs become a part of your life. (The herb profiles in part 3, page 107, include the energetic qualities of each plant.)

In addition, people have a sort of baseline type, called a *constitution*. We all know someone who is quick to blush, perspires easily, and is maybe a little clumsy. We may also know someone who can't put on a pound to save their soul, is constantly cold, and is very tense. Those "types" are not going to change much. Different constitutions typically need to be taken into account when working to return to balance. Someone who is always cold, thin, active, and dry will need warming, relaxing, moistening herbs. Someone more relaxed, warm, and heavy will want the opposite to fight inertia.

In many of the symptoms we'll be looking at in this book, the same remedy will be useful for everyone. In others, we've created remedies in which an herb that might be drying is ameliorated by the addition of something moistening.

Plant medicine can help you move toward balance. You can give plants a hand. The remedies you'll find in this book work with the energetics of the symptom using herbs that are energetically best suited for correcting imbalances in the body that interfere with emotional healing or well-being. The herbs were chosen because they are helpful for everyone. On page 145 in the Herbal Ally Substitutes, you will find a cross-referenced list so that in the event that an herb doesn't agree with you or you can't find it, you can easily find a substitute.

Working with the Root Causes of Imbalance

No matter what happens to you in your emotional life, the stronger your body is, the better you'll be able to maintain balance and rebound from a setback.

For example, when my daughter was born, I was determined to do everything perfectly. I wound up not sleeping more than an hour or two a day, and after six weeks, my postpartum depression was on a fast train to psychosis. One single night of uninterrupted sleep restored me to almost normal, but if I had just stayed healthy physically, I would have been fine emotionally.

Our organs create toxins in order to work, like a car puts out exhaust. If we remain healthy and strong, those waste products are processed and are eliminated through either the bladder, bowel, perspiration, or breathing. If some prankster comes along and puts a potato in the exhaust of a car, it will stop running in short order. When humans can't eliminate their organ-by-product toxins, they can build up and make us weak and vulnerable to not just physical ailments but also emotional, mental, and spiritual problems. In the extreme, those toxins go beyond causing muscular pain and skin outbreaks. They'll accumulate in the brain, causing confusion, hallucinations, coma, and sometimes even death. By any means necessary, if you can prioritize eating well, getting exercise, or practicing some kind of meditation or yoga, you will create a strong foundation to help balance your state of mind.

While herbs can't do it all, they help a lot—and they are so simple to include in your everyday life. Some herbs are just very enjoyable teas, seasonings for your meals, or good at lending luxury and comfort to your bath. You may get to the point where you can't remember life before herbs. They are that easy to incorporate.

HOW ARE YOU DOING TODAY?

Sometimes, when you're in the middle of something, you can't judge things clearly. You may be so accustomed to telling your friends and loved ones that you're fine that you don't pay attention to how you *really* feel. (It's funny how we can so often see what's happening in other people's lives, but in our own it isn't so easy, and we can't see the forest for the trees.) There are some things you can do to try to understand what's going on.

- A journal has always helped me. It's like having a long talk with a friend (which is great, too).
- Keep a list of how you feel, when you feel that way, who was there, what led up to it, and so on. That will let you see patterns.
- It's also really helpful to have imaginary conversations and even arguments when you're alone. Any way that you can express what's inside without judgment may shine a light on what needs work.
- If you can bear what might feel like criticism, ask your loved ones how you're coming across to them.

The signals you might recognize could be a desire to stay home or even in bed, no interest in what is normally exciting, a change in eating habits, or skipping showers. Personally, I notice that the world seems to lose colors and that there isn't much that I find funny. If you knew me, the lack of humor would be a huge tip-off. Are you feeling like yourself?

Complementary Practices to Herbal Medicine

While it may feel like the last thing you can manage, it's important to pay attention to self-care. Keeping up with hygiene, sleep, nutrition, and contact with others can keep us feeling good about ourselves. Here are some suggestions to shift a heavy mood:

- Movement, such as yoga, tai chi, or aerobics, releases endorphins, which are naturally occurring brain chemicals that feel good. If all you feel up for is a short walk, do it; getting your blood flowing can make a huge difference, and you can always build up from there.

- Get a massage, manicure, pedicure, or a new haircut. Massage releases endorphins, lactic acid, and histamines, and drains lymph nodes. Toxins are moved for easier elimination. Human touch is important, too.

- Go outside and hug a tree. Open up and allow the tree to hug you back. Trust me, it's an amazing feeling. Of course, just being out in nature will reduce any physical manifestations of stress and anxiety. If it's warm enough, take off your shoes and feel the earth under your bare feet. This will ground you and remind you that all of nature wants you to feel at peace!

- Eat good food. Hit the produce aisle hard, and avoid processed foods if possible.

- Stay hydrated. The brain is up to 73 percent water, so dehydration gums up the works.

- Be your own friend. One of the kindest things to do for yourself is to keep internal dialogue as gentle as you would if talking to your best friend. We never tell our friends that they are incompetent or unworthy, but somehow we rarely treat ourselves as well.

In addition, there are lots of different complementary or alternative practitioners who can help you clear dense energy and help you to lift out of a dark place. They are all helpful for issues that are physical, emotional, or spiritual.

- Flower essences are used more and more frequently. These essences contain almost no flower/herb but are created in such a way that the plant releases its healing spirit into pure, distilled or spring water, which is then blended with brandy to preserve it. The doses for flower essences are very small; you only need a few drops. When used consistently, you can begin to feel the effects over time. A good practitioner can fine-tune a remedy for any number of emotional issues.

- Reiki practitioners can channel energy that helps clear blockages that weigh us down. That's also something you can learn to do for yourself. The first level, or attunement, of Reiki allows the individual to work on themselves or others. Reiki is very good for physical aches and pains but is also very healing for heartbreak, worry, and many emotional issues.

- Acupuncture or acupressure will also work to clear blocked energy pathways.

- Homeopathy is similar to flower essences but uses different types of plants and sometimes non-plant substances. They are used to address emotional issues, particularly when we are "stuck" and can't move past something.

- Aromatherapy uses essential oils and hydrosols, and we inhale the scents to flip switches in our limbic brains for emotional benefits, while they also contain healing constituents for our physical health.

- Emotional Freedom Technique (EFT) tapping is an easily learned practice that involves clearing meridians by gently tapping specific points in sequence.

- Mindfulness is a practice of learning to stay in the present moment by using breathing, meditation, visualization.

This is but a sampling of ways that can help you feel relaxed, decrease stress—and ultimately find contentment.

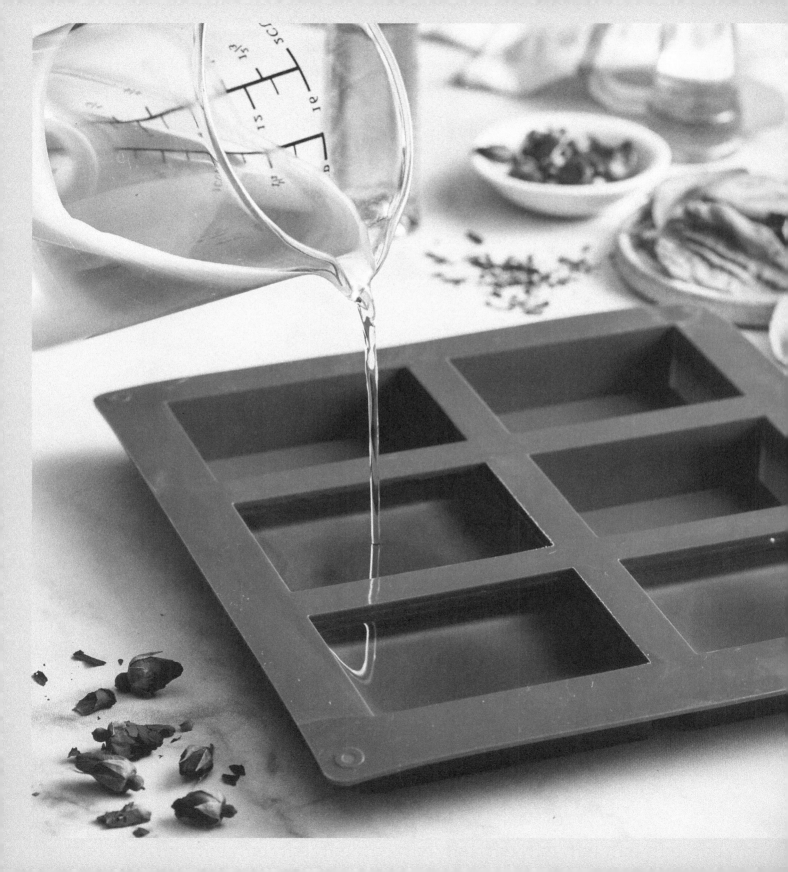

CHAPTER 2

Working with Herbal Medicine

Herbal medicine making is an incredibly fulfilling skill to possess. Before we dig in, there are some details and preparations to think about. How do we choose the right things? What would be the best kind of preparation to create, and what do we need to make that happen? You'll find that there are a lot of things and bits of information that can make the processes easier and less intimidating.

Sourcing Medicinal Plants

Purchasing herbs may seem difficult, but there are a few simple things you can do to ensure that you're getting good-quality plant medicine. The ideal situation is to seek out an herb shop where the person behind the counter knows where the herbs came from and can help you decide. Be aware that, legally, they cannot prescribe or diagnose.

Herb shops aren't always available, but there are some very good places to source herbs online. I recommend that (at least at first) you purchase in smaller quantities, so you can see if the herb is one that works for you. If you have the space, growing herbs is also a fantastic way to access high-quality, fresh herbs, so go for it!

The Resources section (page 151) includes some of my favorite recommendations for herbs, herbal products, and seeds or plants.

Common Preparations to Buy

It's easy to purchase good herbal medicine. In the list that follows, I've provided the most common herbal preparations you can find to buy. I've also marked those that are easy to make at home with an asterisk. (And you can surely make the rest at home, but they may require more instruction, study, or attention to detail.) Whether you purchase or DIY comes down to your budget and how much time, energy, and motivation you've got. When you're feeling blue, it may be easier to purchase your herbs online and have them delivered to your door, and know that's a great option.

- Teas*
- Tinctures* (easy but need to sit for a few weeks)
- Fresh or dried individual herbs
- Syrups*
- Capsules or lozenges
- Balms and salves*
- Lotions
- Soaps
- Bath teas and soaks*
- Elixirs*
- Herbal vinegars* (easy but may need to sit for a few weeks)
- Infused honeys* (easy but may need time to infuse)
- Seasonings for food

Red Flags to Avoid

Steer clear of herbs that have lost their color—and, by extension, their vitality. Dull color indicates that they've been sitting around, and age as well as poor storage practices will diminish the plant's medicinal properties. Never purchase any kind of herbal product from a gas station or convenience store because they're

PROTECTING AT-RISK PLANTS

Years ago, people in rural communities commonly made their livings by foraging and collecting wild plants for drug companies. This is still done, but more herbs are cultivated. However, there are still several plants that thrive and are more potent growing in the wild. These plants face many threats. Loss of habitat, use of herbicides, and fewer and fewer pollinators are part of the problem, and as more people become interested in herbs, overharvesting is a huge issue. Wild ginseng, goldenseal, and trillium are rare sights because they're worth money. Sandalwood and Palo Santo are popular scents, the plants of which are becoming few and far between. Here's how you can help keep these herbal allies from becoming threatened.

- Learn alternatives to at-risk herbs.
- Never use more than you need.
- If you choose to harvest a wild plant, take no more than 10 percent of a stand, leaving seeds behind. If there is only one stand, take nothing.
- Consider planting some endangered plants on your property to replace what you use.
- Join and contribute to United Plant Savers (unitedplantsavers.org) to be aware of the plants that are at risk.

There are people who still sell these plants and products made from them. Do not hesitate to ask about the origin. As an example, white sage is at risk, so I grow it and distill it for the hydrosol, taking nothing from the wild. There will be times when it is reasonable to use one of these herbs, but be mindful of their status, and buy or use only what you really need. Don't waste it. It is so much better to learn about and use plants that are growing abundantly around you.

selling a trend and don't know anything about it. Instead, go directly to herb sellers who are only working with herbs and herbal products rather than unfamiliar, random web stores. See the Resources section (page 151) for good sources.

Best Practices and Safety Precautions

A safe and respectful approach to herbal medicine will lead to rich and fulfilling experiences.

Best Practices

I've learned the following best practices and found that they make herbalism feel like a lifestyle. (Which, as you may be coming to realize, it is!)

- Choose one herb when there is no urgent need to use it, and really get to know it. Note how it makes you feel. Then do the same with another single herb. That way you can begin to understand how herbs affect you. If you make or buy a blend and then have a reaction, there's no way to know which herb caused it. If the blend works like magic, again, it will be a mystery. As you find your own allies, it will be easier and easier to discern what you need.

- Find a few people nearby who are interested in learning about herbs. Gather in

a kitchen and try blending teas, making salves, or whatever you've been wanting to try. Take field guides out into the woods and work together to identify plants. Each person brings some knowledge whether they know it or not, and it's fun. Join some online groups and learn from the discussions. I still learn new things all the time from both of those sources.

- Make small batches of herbal medicine. I love to make 4-ounce batches of tinctures when working with a new herb and never make more than a pint. An ounce or two of a tea blend is usually plenty.

- Choose a preparation that you will actually use. Something that sits in a jar because it's unpleasant to take isn't helping at all. Capsules get a pretty bad rap because herbs are thought to be more easily absorbed in teas, tinctures, vinegars, and the like, but for many people, they're the most convenient method of taking herbs. The best way to take herbs is the way *you* will actually take them. They only work if they are used.

- If an herb shop salesperson attempts to add several more products to your purchase, be wary. Herbs can get expensive. It's frustrating to have a cupboard full of bottles and jars that didn't work and cost a paycheck. Instead, get one or two items at a time unless a practitioner has recommended them. Keep in mind that in medicine, pharmacists don't diagnose or prescribe, and physicians don't sell drugs. That is to protect patients and consumers. The lines aren't that clear in herbalism, so it's something to consider.

Safety Precautions

Before long, working safely with herbs will become second nature, but here are some tips to help you establish good habits:

- Always label everything. You will not remember what's in that amber bottle next spring, and you will need to throw it out, and that is very sad. There is a bottle of tincture and a jar of some kind of infused oil downstairs right now that I have to throw out for this very reason. (Yes, I still overestimate my memory sometimes.) Labeling for personal use should include the ingredients, the date, what it is, and why it was made.

- Wash bottles and jars in hot soapy water prior to use. Running them through the dishwasher is great, too.

- Small batches mean that there is less chance of spoilage. It's better to make enough for a week or two and then make it again than to make too much and have it go bad. Alcohol and vinegar are very good preservatives, so products made with them are very safe, but it is still best to use them up.

- Just because herbs are natural, it doesn't mean they are harmless—if they weren't powerful, they couldn't help you! Less is usually more, so work up to larger doses. Be sure of the herb. It's always good to check more than one source of information.

- Honey, especially raw honey—which is generally preferred—should not be given to children younger than one year old. Their digestive systems are not mature enough to process Clostridium, a bacteria often found in honey that can turn into botulism in infants.

Tools, Equipment, and Ingredients

Happily, there are very few things needed that you don't already have in the kitchen. Over the years I've accumulated some really cool herb tools, but they arrived either as gifts or from a yard sale or thrift store. The hunt was half the fun! Some people enjoy going all out and getting the fancy equipment, but it can also be done inexpensively.

Essential Tools and Equipment

I started on a shoestring and can honestly say that with a whisk, measuring spoons and cups, a tea strainer, and some jars, it is possible to make just about everything you'll find in this book. There are some other items that come in handy and make the process more enjoyable, and it's much easier to work with some good tools.

- Whisk to combine wet or dry ingredients

- Containers: jars, bottles, and waterproof bag (feel free to reuse all glass bottles and jars of a reasonable size; just wash and sterilize them first)

- Fine-mesh strainer or 8-inch to 12-inch squares of cloth from worn-out T-shirts, sheets, or flannel

- Mixing bowls in a few different sizes or a 1- or 2-quart glass measuring cup

- A few dark glass dropper bottles in various sizes—1-ounce, 2-ounce, and 4-ounce—to hold finished and strained liquids

- Small jars for salves and lip balms

- Labels

- Permanent marker: something that won't smudge if it gets wet

Some other items that are quite possibly already in your kitchen or that you will want to keep an eye out for as your herbal adventures continue:

- Coffee grinder for powdering herbs (a mortar and pestle may look cool, but the coffee grinder will save you time and your wrists)

- 5-by-8-inch muslin bags: great for making half gallons of tea or straining tinctures or oils

- Electric teapot to heat water quickly (I use mine nearly every day)

- 1-quart slow cooker: good for decoctions of roots and barks for tea or for infusing oils

- Blender: helps combine any sort of dry ingredients or chops up fresh herbs for tincturing

- Pipettes: long, disposable droppers

Helpful Ingredients

The following items will show up in the recipes that follow in part 2. If there's something you don't have, you should be able to find a different remedy that uses other ingredients, so don't worry if you haven't got everything. There will be lots of choices for you.

The good news is that most of the ingredients are available at the grocery or liquor store. Here's what you'll be using in addition to herbs:

- Alcohol, 100-proof vodka or 151-proof grain alcohol: used to make tinctures

- Apple cider vinegar: can be infused with herbs and used either internally or externally

- Coconut oil: can be infused for internal or external applications

- Epsom salt: makes a wonderfully soothing bath ingredient when mixed with herbs

- Honey: sweetens teas and also is a good preservative and thickener

- Oatmeal: is excellent in the bath or as a facial scrub

- Olive oil: can be infused with herbs and soothe sore or injured skin

- Powdered milk: this goes into the tub (it can be any kind as long as it's powdered)

- Rice: is a nice weight when added to a pouch that can be heated and applied to sore muscles

- Witch hazel: makes a good liniment base

These two items are useful, but they're not usually available except in herb shops or craft stores. Check the Resources section (page 151) for sources.

- Glycerin: can be used to make tinctures when alcohol is not a good option

- Beeswax: used in any kind of balm or salve to thicken to the proper consistency

Dosages and Protocols

Most of us are accustomed to using pharmaceutical medications. Even though many of those drugs are derived from herbs, they are specific components of the herbs. We take the whole herb, meaning that we get the protections and buffers that naturally occur in the plants. This also means that

- It may take longer to feel a difference.

- Herbs are much gentler.

- There is less chance for side effects.

- The dosage is not nearly as critical as with pharmaceutical drugs.

I should mention that it it's not unusual for me to feel almost instant relief from herbs meant to help me relax or leave the black clouds behind. Most herbs work pretty quickly for me, but everyone has different results and responses.

Dosage Recommendations

In this book, we'll be focusing on very safe herbs, and for the most part, overuse may only result in mild intestinal discomfort or diarrhea. There are very few hard-and-fast rules about dosages regarding herbs, but the best rule is to start with the smallest dose and work up. For very young children, a tiny bit goes a long way. When my daughter was a toddler, we'd have a tea party using herbal tea, or I'd put one or two drops of tincture into her juice. Those who are pregnant or nursing can partake of many herbs, especially in moderation; after all, we use them to season our foods all the time. However, there are some that stimulate the uterus or pass through to the mother's milk (which is sometimes very handy), so pay attention to any warnings.

Unlike the way drugs are titrated to weight, herbs work differently for different people. They teach you to pay attention and listen to your body. Since we've been conditioned to ignore many of our body's signals, it may be a bit difficult to detect at first. It's good to keep a journal or notebook where you can jot down how you feel.

Practical Protocols

Although you'll receive guidelines with each recipe, they are only guidelines. Here are some things to keep in mind:

- It's best to start small with internal preparations (such as infusions, teas, tinctures, etc.) and pay close attention for any reaction, like allergies (pretty rare) or diarrhea or constipation (not so rare).

- Most herbs taken for a condition work best if taken 2 to 4 times a day. This depends on the herb, the condition, and your constitution. In order to gauge whether it is the right herb, you need to take it regularly for at least a week or more depending on the purpose. Just like pharmaceuticals, they all work differently—and at their own pace.

- If you are working with herbal allies for physical conditions, it depends on the severity of the issue, but in general, you should see an improvement within a week

or two. Anything that shows worsening or infection is a signal to get help.

- Know when to seek help. Right now you're in need of emotional wellness, so if your sadness increases or you have trouble telling what's real and begin to hallucinate, it is time to see your doctor. If you start having thoughts of harming yourself or others, seek help immediately. (See page 152 for the suicide prevention hotline number.)

- Pay attention to suggestions from loved ones. We hate to hear that we are overreacting or acting unlike our usual selves, but the people who love us often see it before we do. If a week or two go by and there's no improvement, consider talking to your family physician or a therapist.

The Importance in Seeking Help
There's no shame in deciding that it's time to see a physician, psychologist, or psychiatrist. The important thing is to get better. That doesn't negate the herbal experience, and all the different modalities of wellness can get along just fine. It is important to let doctors know exactly what herbs have been taken.

Substituting Herbal Allies

In the '90s, my sister and I had an herb shop, and we gave weekly classes on all kinds of herbal things. We learned that no matter what we taught, it was hard for some people to feel comfortable expanding on or changing the recipe. That was something we really tried to stress, though, because flexibility is part of the beauty of herbs. One herb may be the perfect choice for me but have the opposite effect on you. For instance, chamomile is a favorite relaxing cup of tea for me, but it may make someone else sneeze or get itchy.

You'll find an Herbal Ally Substitutes chart on page 145 to help you make substitutions from among the herbs we're using in the recipes in part 2.

If you're just starting out with herbs, this may be hard to believe, but the fact is that if just 5 or 10 herbs resonate with you and you learn as much as you can about them, it will be no time at all before you are creating your own recipes and making substitutions without stressing about it in the least.

I've noticed that in some herb groups (for instance, the Herb Society of America), members take turns researching a particular herb, writing a three- to four-page report, and then presenting it to the group. They make several things, like a tea blend, cookies that include the herb, and a salve or syrup to share at the meeting. It can be a great source of information. The key is to get to know each ally. Prepare it different ways so you can drink it, eat it, bathe in it, and so on. Discover how it makes you feel in different preparations. Then you'll feel secure that you know the herb well.

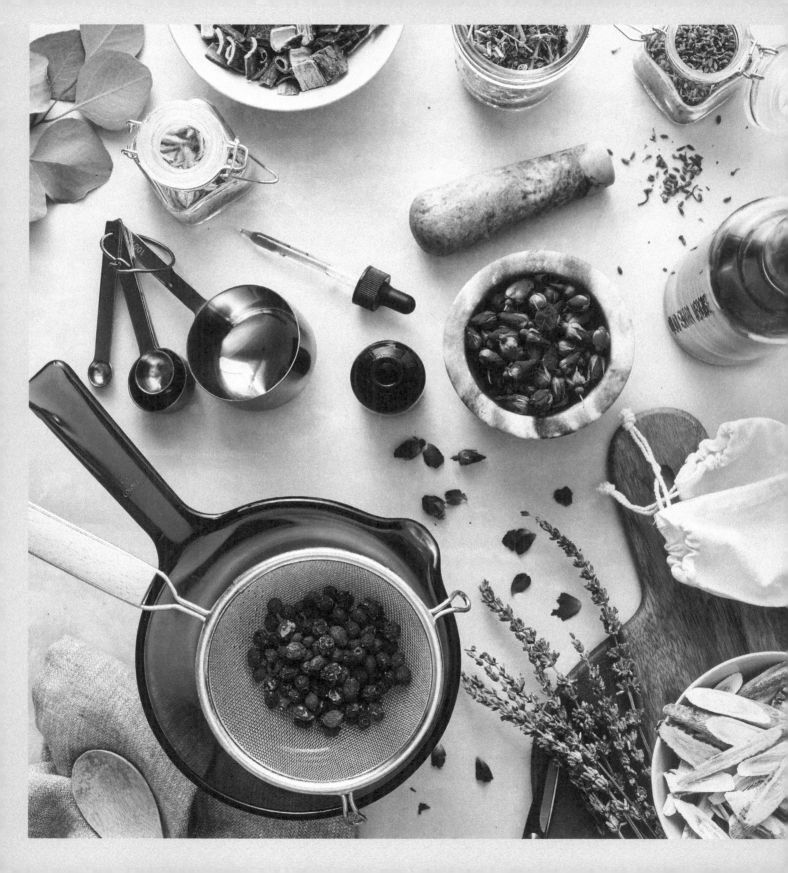

CHAPTER 3

Herbal Preparations for Emotional Well-Being

When you're feeling emotionally raw, you may not have the motivation or energy to gather lots of kitchen supplies and ingredients to prepare a complicated herbal remedy. That's why I've kept most of the herbal preparations in this book straight-forward. And fortunately, some of the most potent ways to ingest herbs are also the simplest. You may choose to make some ahead of time (like a tincture, which comes together quickly but needs weeks of macerating time) or create them on the spur of the moment as needed (like a simple tea). Knowing how to make them can bolster your confidence and sometimes provide stillness in a storm.

This chapter provides an overview of the various types of herbal preparations you'll find in part 2 (page 29), from the easiest to the hardest.

Teas

Teas are about the gentlest way to partake of herbal medicine. Almost all of us have enjoyed a cup of chamomile or mint tea without even realizing we were drinking a tea with medicinal properties. In fact, black tea and coffee are medicinal, too.

A "tisane" refers to a tea that contains no *Camellia sinensis*, true tea. It can be any plant, root, leaf, flower, seed, or blend of any of these. You'll discover many beneficial blends in part 2.

To brew a cup of herbal tea, measure out about a teaspoon of herbs to 6 ounces of water (for stronger effects, the quantity of herbs can be doubled or more). Bring your water just to a boil, and then add it to your mug with the loose herbs or tea infuser.

- You can easily get by with a small pan to heat water and a fine-mesh strainer to remove the herbs from the water.

- A tea kettle and one of the many types of infusers make it easier but aren't necessary.

- Herb tea can stay in the cup while it is drunk and not get bitter like regular black tea does. Instead of needing to remove the herb tea bag after a few minutes as with black tea, herb teas just get better.

- Honey makes the perfect sweetener if desired.

- Tea can be prepared ahead, refrigerated, and reheated or enjoyed cold, if that's easier. I make teas by the gallon several times a week and drink them cold.

- Be aware of side effects of the herbs in your tea and drink accordingly. The last thing you want is for the herbs to make you feel worse than you already do.

Decoctions

Decoctions resemble teas but are used for barks, seeds, and roots, which take a little more time and heat to extract their healing properties into the water. Barks like mimosa and roots like ashwagandha, astragalus, echinacea, and licorice roots are decocted. They can also be decocted into other liquids, like vinegar and oil, but the term is used almost exclusively with water as the menstruum (what we call the liquid/solvent in which the herbs soak). Higher heat is used, and the decoction is boiled or simmered until the marc (or herb) has clearly released its properties into the water, which is reduced to a much stronger drink than tea. You'll know decoction is taking place by the way it looks, smells, and tastes.

- Use a heavy saucepan (or stockpot for large batches).

- Heat to a simmer and hold there for between 30 and 60 minutes.

- Add water as necessary to keep the herbs in liquid.

- Store any unused decoction in the refrigerator for up to 5 days.

- Decoctions can be added to infusions. For instance, to a cup of mint tea you could add 1 tablespoon of echinacea decoction for an immunity boost. Or you could add a splash of mimosa bark decoction to a cup of holy basil tea to brighten the day.

- Pay attention to how much you drink, as these are more concentrated. If there are side effects, they will occur more readily than with a tea.

Tinctures

Tinctures are my favorite way to preserve herbs, and they're very easy to make—and take, too. If you're newer to herbs, they might not be familiar and may seem a little mysterious, but they're so easy! A tincture is made by soaking herbs in alcohol for a period of time, during which the medicinal properties of the herbs are transferred into the alcohol. A very general way of looking at it is that a dropperful (which is 25 to 30 drops) is about equivalent to a cup of tea made from the herb. This is a very efficient means of taking a dose of herbs.

If using alcohol is not an option for you, you can substitute vegetable glycerin. This is called a "glycerite" or "glycerin tincture," and the menstruum is made up of 3 parts glycerin and 1 part water. Glycerites aren't quite as effective, and they don't last as long

as alcohol-based tinctures, but for children or adults who don't want to use alcohol, glycerites are a great option. The easiest way of making tinctures is the "folk method," in which eyeballing the herbs and menstruum trumps using precise measurements.

Here's another great use for those jars you've been saving:

- If using dried herbs, fill your jar (any size) between ⅓ and ½ full.

- If using fresh herbs, chop and loosely fill the jar.

- Cover the herbs with the menstruum.

- They will remain in the jar, soaking, for between two and six weeks. Strain and transfer into dropper bottles. Glycerites have a shorter shelf life (6 months to a year), so strain them and keep them handy so they are used. Alcohol tinctures stay active almost indefinitely.

- It's really nice to have some dropper bottles to use with tinctures, but ¼ and ½ teaspoon measuring spoons work as well.

To take tinctures, it's easiest to mix them with a little water or juice. I often put them into a cup of tea. Some people take them straight, but there's no need for that. The exception would be if you're taking bitters for digestion; then it is important to taste them. Glycerites are sweet and a bit thick, so kids usually don't mind them.

For little ones, try a drop per age up until about 12 years of age. The herbs you'll explore in this book can all be taken by adults at a dose of about 25 to 30 drops, which is about a dropperful.

Elixirs and Tonics

Elixirs and tonics are fanciful old-fashioned names for preparations that are a lot like tinctures but are combinations of alcohol, vinegar, honey, and herbs.

An elixir is made by mixing both alcohol and honey in varying proportions with the marc. Rose elixir is usually made with glycerin, and since it's already sweet, it's just touched with honey. Because they are sweet, elixirs can be taken by the spoonful, like a syrup.

A tonic can really be almost anything. It might be part alcohol tincture, part herb vinegar, and another part honey, and maybe the honey was infused with an herb. There might be some decoction mixed in there, too. Tonics usually include several different herbs and/or roots. The term "tonic" is used to convey the idea that it is taken on a long-term basis to tone or improve your health in some way. Tonics are usually not used for acute conditions.

Baths and Soaks

There are times when water comes and washes away our worries, stress, pain, and restlessness. It may be in the form of an infusion for the tub or a nice soothing hand or foot soak. It forces you to slow down for a moment and lets you collect your thoughts. Adding herbs to your soaking water layers the experience, soothing the skin and providing a mild aromatherapy effect. I like to imagine any sadness or negativity being drawn from my body, swirling in the water—and down the drain. The warmth of the water can also make it easier to drift off to sleep.

Bath teas and soaks are very much like teas that you drink, and in fact there are some that you may enjoy sipping while bathing. Herbs and additives such as oatmeal, salt, or powdered milk are mixed together. In order to really release the properties into the water effectively, use a 1-gallon heat-resistant pitcher to make a strong tea while the tub fills. That gallon of tea is then added to the bath along with the package of herbs.

These blends can be prepared in a reasonable quantity so they are ready when needed. Large heat-sealable tea bags and large muslin drawstring bags make it possible to portion them into individual baths/soaks so that they take barely any thought at all.

Bath teas that do not include oatmeal, milk, or salts can be used in Jacuzzi tubs if you have access to one. In that case, leave the herbal package out of the tub; just pour the hot tea into the tub.

You'll find several lovely bathing herbs and soaks in part 2 (page 29).

Infused Herbal Honey

Herbal honeys are particularly nice for herbs that are not all that tasty or that you'd want to add to any cup of tea. The honey is an effective preservative.

To make infused honey:

- Warm the honey in a heavy pan, low and slow.

- Add 1 part herbs to 3 parts honey.

- Mix well and continue warming covered for an hour or so.

- While the honey is still warm, strain out the herbs.

- Pour into jars.

- Label and date.

For stronger flavor, allow the herbs and honey to steep overnight or even for a couple of days. Just reheat enough to easily strain. This can be done with many herbs.

Infusions

The word "infusion" can mean several things. For our purposes here, it means using various liquids other than water or alcohol, to which you'll add dried herbs for a period of time to infuse the liquid (or menstruum) with the properties of the herbs (or marc). Most of the time, oil, vinegar, or solid fats can be infused.

You might opt to infuse vinegar with nettle to extract the plants' abundant minerals and nutrients, or you may infuse oil with soothing or circulatory herbs to make a muscle rub.

To make a vinegar infusion:

- Fill a glass jar ½ full with dried herbs (or nearly full with fresh herbs) and cover with vinegar, tucking any stray bits of herb under the surface. Cover with either a plastic lid or a metal lid lined with parchment paper before closing the jar. The vinegar can be strained and used within a few days if necessary, but it's best to leave it to infuse for two weeks, if possible.

To make an oil infusion:

- If using dried herbs, follow the preceding instructions.

- If using fresh herbs:

  ◆ Wilt the herbs overnight to remove excess moisture.

  ◆ You *can* infuse them in a warm, dry place for two weeks, keeping a close eye for any herbs above the surface (which will quickly mold), or, if you want them sooner, you can put the wilted herbs and oil into a mini slow cooker for about 4 hours. The slow cooker method can be used for dried herbs, too. No slow cooker? Put the herbs and oil in a deep enough baking pan and place them in the oven set on "warm" for several hours.

The oil or vinegar is then strained and kept in a cool, dark place until needed. If you don't foresee yourself using it in a couple of weeks, refrigerate the oil. Vinegars do not require refrigeration, but some people prefer to keep them refrigerated, and that's fine, too.

- Glass jars are perfect for this, so if you've been saving them, you're ready.

- The infusion should take place without a lid. If a lid is used on the finished vinegar, be sure it isn't metal or line it with parchment paper.

- A small slow cooker is nice, but the oven works just as well.

- I've tried coffee filters and cheesecloth, but fabric squares saved from worn clothing or sheets works best for straining the herbs from your infusion.

- It's best to use dry herbs with oil. Fresh herbs contain water, which can cause mold, so if using fresh, let your herbs wilt at least overnight. The heating should take care of it, but then store the finished product in the fridge. Pour off any moisture that forms on the top of the oil that will solidify in the cold.

Balms, Salves, and Lotion Bars

The basic concept of balms and salves involves using a combination of oil and (usually) beeswax. There are vegetable waxes that can be used, and some oils are solid and don't require anything to make them harder. We've all used some form of these preparations. Maybe your mom used a mentholated salve on your chests when you were little or you've slathered your lips with lip balm in the winter to heal chapping. There are many, many ways to enjoy them.

Oils are infused with herbs for various purposes and sometimes essential oils to create something special.

One of the main differences between the various types of these preparations is the amount of wax to oil.

Here are some guidelines:

1 part wax to 8 parts infused oil = very soft and loose salve
1 part wax to 4 parts infused oil = a stiffer balm, the hardness of lip balm
1 part wax to 2 parts infused oil = lotion bar hardness

- If it turns out too hard, gently heat and add oil.

- If it is too loose, gently heat and add wax.

- Instead of heating all the oil to a temperature high enough to melt the wax, I find it easier to heat a small amount (¼ to ⅓) of the oil, melt the wax in that, and then gradually add the rest of the oil while still on the heat. If the oil is added too quickly, the wax immediately hardens and doesn't combine with the wax, and then the whole thing has to be reheated. This allows the mixture to cool and set up more quickly.

- Many people choose to use double boilers to heat the oil because it is slower. Other people choose to heat it in the micro-wave using 30-second increments. We are making very small batches, and in the amount of time required to make them, the oil will not scorch or burn if we use the warm setting on the stove. All of these methods are acceptable, so do what is comfortable for you. Just be sure to heat the mixture gently.

- To reduce greasiness, add a pinch of cornstarch. Only a pinch.

- Make small batches. 4 ounces of a salve can last a long time.

- Olive oil is the easiest to obtain, so we'll be using that. It lasts about a year.

- When the scent of the balm changes and becomes slightly unpleasant, discon-tinue use and throw it away. It's time to make more!

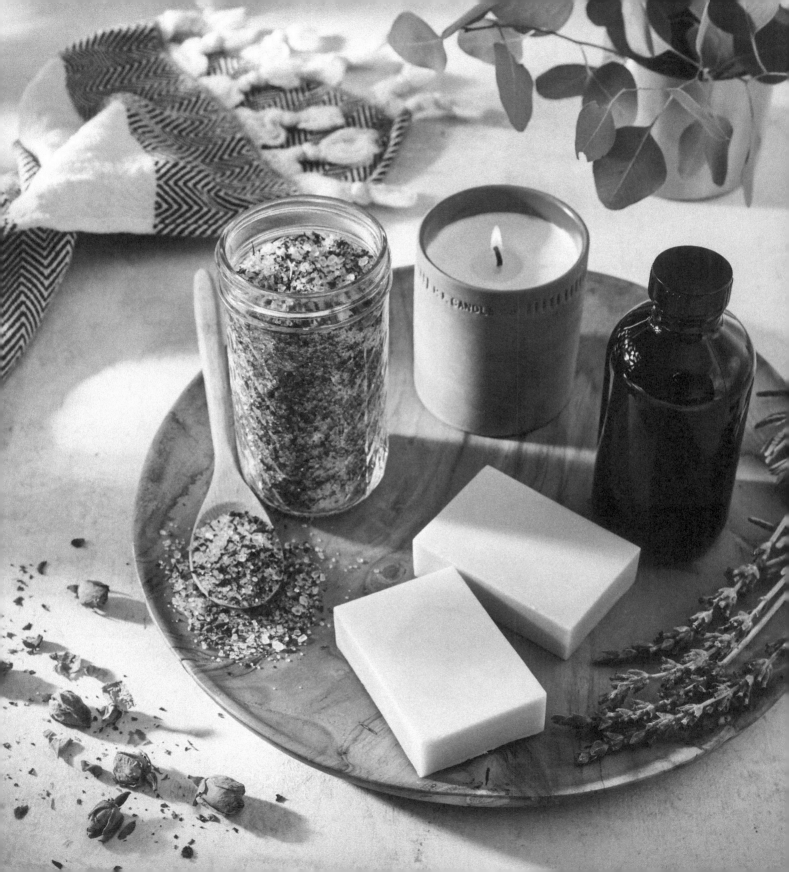

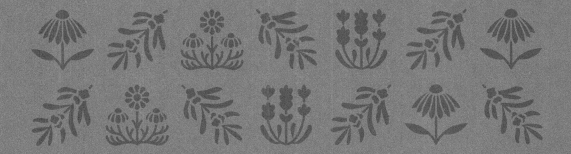

PART TWO

Remedies to Support Emotional Healing

In this part, you'll find descriptions of several common emotional conditions and a wide range of symptoms associated with those conditions. These are followed by recipes for herbal preparations that may help support or relieve these symptoms. Many of these remedies can assist with more than one symptom or emotional condition, so feel free to experiment to discover which work best for you.

A few things to note about the recipes: All recipes for combination tinctures (or oils) can be made from a combination of single tinctures (or oils), or you can blend the herbs together to create your combination tincture (or oil). The following recipes all call for dried herbs unless otherwise noted.

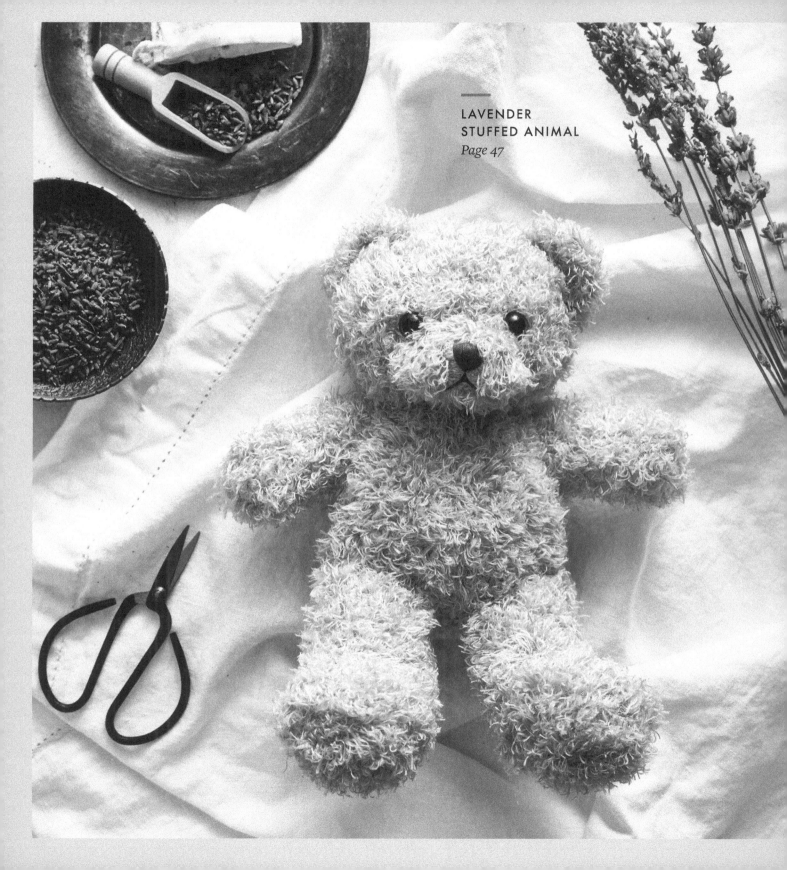

LAVENDER
STUFFED ANIMAL
Page 47

CHAPTER 4
Anxiety

Anxiety can be mild—or it can be a raging monster that wrecks everything in its path. It can build upon itself and make us feel powerless to help ourselves. Anxiety shows up in lots of different ways, and while a few of them can be helpful and motivate us, most of them actually hold us back. Like many mental and emotional conditions, anxiety can create a lot of physical manifestations and can even threaten our spiritual lives, leading us to question beliefs and thoughts. Herbs can be a big help in rounding the rough corners of anxiety.

Anger

This is a hot and tense condition, so the focus, constitutionally, is to cool down and soothe that tension. There are many ways anger is expressed. It took me 40 years to learn how to let it out in a healthy way. Waiting until it boils over is not productive, and it also takes a toll on our organs. There are herbs that can ease that transition from teeth-gritting, fist-clenching anger to something a little less out of control. Occasionally, just being aware of how much anger you're holding and doing something to harness it can start the shift.

Anger Chaser Tincture
MAKES 2 OUNCES

We all have felt angry, and it's often something we try to hide or feel ashamed of feeling. I suppose that in order for all of us to live together in a peaceable society, we've made anger into an emotion that shouldn't be expressed, making it all the more difficult to handle. This soothing herbal blend can help cool things down.

3 tablespoons blue vervain tincture

3 tablespoons skullcap tincture

2 tablespoons mimosa tincture

1. In a measuring cup, combine the blue vervain, skullcap, and mimosa tinctures.

2. Transfer the mixture into a 2-ounce dropper bottle.

3. Label and date the tincture blend.

4. Take 1 dropperful (25 to 30 drops) in 1 ounce of water or juice. Repeat the dose 30 minutes later if needed.

5. Store the tincture blend in a cool, dark place, where it will last for several years.

Misophonia Honey Electuary
MAKES ABOUT 6 OUNCES

The term "misophonia" may be unfamiliar, but it's shocking how many people have it. It is when the sounds that people make eating, clearing their throats, clicking a pen, or humming or other innocent sounds incur a rage that is beyond reason. It sounds like no big deal unless you have it. It is painful, scary, and infuriating, and it is a symptom of chronic anxiety. This sweet herbal paste is easy to take along with you as you go about your day and can either be eaten or added to hot water for an instant tea.

4 tablespoons holy basil

4 tablespoons lemon balm

2 tablespoons motherwort

¾ cup honey

1. In a coffee grinder, working one herb at a time, powder the holy basil, lemon balm, and motherwort. Sift the herbs

through a mesh strainer to remove bits of stem and transfer to a bowl.

2. Add the honey to the powdered herb mixture 1 ounce at a time, until the mixture forms a thick paste. Use more honey if you prefer a thinner mixture.

3. Transfer to a 6-ounce jar or a combination of smaller jars.

4. Label and date the electuary.

5. Add ½ to 1 teaspoon to hot water to make tea or eat off a spoon up to 3 times a day.

6. Refrigerate the electuary and use within a month. (It'll likely keep for much longer, but I've never had them last that long!)

Tip: To preserve the blend longer, decrease the honey by about 2 tablespoons so the mixture forms a stiff dough. Roll the dough into "snakes" ½-inch in diameter or smaller and cut into ½-inch pieces. Air-dry them and they'll keep for about a year at room temperature in an airtight container.

Anticipation Support

By some definitions, the difference between anxiety and stress is that anxiety is related to anticipation and stress is more in the present. Generally speaking, most of the things we worry about don't happen, or they're not as bad as we'd expected. Unfortunately, anxiety doesn't care how many times things turn out fine. Anxiety works to remind us of all the things that could go wrong.

Cool-It Tincture
MAKES 4 OUNCES

The cooling nervines in this tincture blend can transform edgy, wiry energy into something smoother and a little mellower. It's perfect for the type of feeling when something is supposed to happen or isn't on time and someone says, "calm down," not knowing how close they came to getting smacked. I'm not sure why anyone ever says such an unhelpful thing to someone who is upset. As always, breathe. This is also a very nice bedtime blend.

3 tablespoons skullcap tincture

2 tablespoons chamomile tincture

2 tablespoons California poppy tincture

1 tablespoon lemon balm tincture

1. In a measuring cup, combine the skullcap, California poppy, chamomile, and lemon balm tinctures.

2. Transfer the mixture into a 4-ounce dropper bottle.

3. Label and date the tincture blend.

4. Take 1 dropperful (25 to 30 drops) in 1 ounce of water or juice up to 4 times a day.

CONTINUES →

5. Store the tincture blend in a cool, dark place, where it will last for several years.

Tip: These measurements are not critical, so don't worry if you go over or under, especially if you opt to make a blended tincture (in which you combine the dried herbs together in the jar of alcohol) rather than using premade singles.

Nerve Support Elixir
MAKES 6 OUNCES

This elixir combines herbs that address more acute nervous upsets and go on to support and nourish nerves to increase resilience.

2 tablespoons skullcap	2 tablespoons milky oats
2 tablespoons motherwort	⅓ cup honey
2 tablespoons chamomile	½ cup alcohol (vodka, rum, or any alcohol of choice)
2 tablespoons astragalus	

1. In a medium (at least 8-ounce) jar, combine the dried skullcap, motherwort, chamomile, astragalus, and milky oats.

2. Add the honey until the jar is about ⅓ full, using a knife to mix it with the herbs.

3. Fill the rest of the jar with your alcohol of choice. Cover the jar and shake well.

4. Infuse the elixir for 2 to 4 weeks, storing it in a cool, dark place and shaking occasionally.

5. Once it's done infusing, strain the elixir and transfer it to a 6-ounce dropper bottle.

6. Label and date the elixir.

7. Take 1 dropperful (25 to 30 drops) each morning and/or evening as needed.

8. Store the elixir in a cool, dark place, where it will last for several years.

Tip: Measurements of the honey and alcohol will vary depending on the size of jar you use. Use the ingredients list as a rough guideline.

Before-the-Storm Nerve Tonic Oxymel
MAKES 16 OUNCES

An oxymel is very much like an elixir, but you replace the alcohol with apple cider vinegar. This blend combines adaptogens, which are herbs that specifically help your body adapt to and manage stress. It calms and supports the nervous system and can be used on a regular basis.

2 tablespoons ashwagandha root	2 tablespoons holy basil
2 tablespoons astragalus root	2 tablespoons eleuthero root
2 tablespoons lemon balm	½ cup honey
2 tablespoons chamomile	2 cups apple cider vinegar

1. In a 1-quart jar with a wide mouth, combine the ashwagandha, astragalus, lemon balm, chamomile, holy basil, and eleuthero.

2. Add the honey and stir with a long spoon to combine with the herbs.

3. Add the vinegar and mix well.

4. If possible, cover with a plastic lid. (If only metal is available, top the jar with a square of parchment paper before securing to prevent the metal lid from rusting.)

5. Infuse the oxymel for 2 to 4 weeks, storing it in a cool, dark place and shaking occasionally.

6. Once it's done infusing, strain the oxymel and transfer it to a bottle.

7. Label and date the oxymel.

8. Add about 1 tablespoon to 4 ounces of water or juice and drink daily.

9. Store in a cool, dry place out of direct sunlight, where it will last for about 1 year.

> **Tip:** When straining out your oxymel, some of the liquid will be lost, as the herbs absorb it, so expect to yield between 16 and 18 ounces.

Body Aches and Muscle Tension

The unrelenting tension of anxiety can result in a body full of aches and pains. Now, on top of feeling emotionally pained, the body acts up. We may be chilled due to blood being called to the trunk and away from the extremities, which only makes things worse. Your herbal allies will help you relax and release that tension. Warmth and herbs work together to relieve the pain.

Everything Hurts Bath Blend
MAKES ENOUGH FOR 4 BATHS

Very warm water, the scent of the herbs, magnesium from the Epsom salt, and the anti-inflammatory toning qualities of witch hazel all combine to make this bath very soothing! Carve out 15 to 20 minutes to yourself, add some pleasant music, and you just may feel like a new person when you emerge from the tub. Have clean pajamas and a warm robe waiting.

1 cup peppermint

1 cup lavender

½ cup rosemary

1½ cups Epsom salt

4 pint bottles witch hazel

1. In a large jar, combine the peppermint, lavender, rosemary, and Epsom salt.

CONTINUES →

2. Add 1 cup of the herb-salt mixture to a washcloth and tie it off. Add it to a bowl of very hot water to brew a strong tea. In the meantime, draw the bath.

3. Once the tub is full, add the hot tea along with the loose herb-salt mixture from the washcloth into the tub. The washcloth full of herbs can be used to gently rinse the body or can be rubbed on sore muscles.

4. Add 1 pint bottle of witch hazel.

5. Sink into the bath and relax for up to 20 minutes.

6. Store the remaining bath blend in an airtight container, where it should keep for a year.

7. Label and date the bath blend.

Tip: Keep individual pint bottles of witch hazel on hand for bathing.

Achy Breaky Tincture
MAKES 2 OUNCES

There are times when everything feels tight and fragile. Sometimes it's hard to even pinpoint the pain because it is diffuse and seems to be everywhere. That's achy breaky. In addition to easing pain, this tincture will probably cause drowsiness, so only take it when it's safe to doze off.

1 tablespoon blue vervain tincture	1 tablespoon St. John's wort tincture
1 tablespoon California poppy tincture	1 tablespoon valerian tincture

1. In a measuring cup, combine the blue vervain, California poppy, St. John's wort, and valerian tinctures.

2. Transfer the mixture into a 2-ounce dropper bottle.

3. Label and date the tincture blend.

4. Take 1 dropperful (25 to 30 drops) in 1 ounce of water or juice. Repeat the dose 30 minutes later if needed.

5. Store the tincture blend in a cool, dark place, where it will last for several years.

Tip: To make this more of a daytime remedy, leave out the California poppy and replace it with catnip.

Sore Muscle Salve
MAKES 4 OUNCES

Tight muscles knot, hurt, and can eventually start to spasm if you ignore the pain. One wrong move and your neck, lower back, or calf muscle clenches and messes up your whole day. It's much better to be aware of your body's needs and respond during the early stages with this terrific, soothing salve.

2½ tablespoons
St. John's wort–infused
olive oil

2 tablespoons
peppermint-infused
olive oil

2½ tablespoons
ginger-infused olive oil

1 tablespoon beeswax
pastilles

1. In a measuring cup, combine the St. John's wort–, ginger-, and peppermint-infused olive oils.

2. In a small pan, combine 2 tablespoons of the oil blend and the beeswax.

3. Heat the mixture slowly until the beeswax liquefies. If using a microwave, heat in 30-second increments and stir well in between. Add the remaining oil blend to the warmed beeswax mixture and stir well to combine.

4. Pour into a 4-ounce jar while still warm and liquid.

5. Label and date the salve.

6. Store the salve in a cool, dry place out of direct sunlight, where it will keep for 6 months.

Tip: This is great to use after an Everything Hurts bath (page 35).

Circulation

The tension of anxiety does a lot of things we don't realize. Our hands and feet are cold, and no amount of rubbing them together or blowing on them helps. We may look down and notice our arms and legs have a vaguely mottled appearance. Anxiety causes our hearts to beat harder and can result in constriction of the vessels.

Cold Hands, Warm Heart Tea Blend

15 (1-CUP) SERVINGS

The following tea not only has warming and relaxing properties, it's also beneficial for your heart and circulatory system.

¼ cup hawthorn berries, leaves, and twigs

2 tablespoons ginger root, chopped small

¼ cup ginkgo leaves

Honey (optional)

¼ cup chamomile

Lemon (optional)

2 tablespoons thyme

1. In a large bowl, combine the hawthorn, ginkgo, chamomile, thyme, and ginger.

2. Transfer the tea blend to an airtight container. Label and date the blend.

3. To use, add 1 rounded teaspoon to an infuser and place in a 10-ounce mug.

4. Cover with just-boiled water and steep for 5 to 7 minutes. Remove the infuser.

5. Sweeten with honey and lemon (if using).

6. Wrap hands around the warm mug and enjoy up to 3 times a day.

CONTINUES →

7. Store in a cool, dry place out of direct sunlight. This will keep for a year.

Cold Hands, Warm Heart Tincture
MAKES 4 OUNCES

You can very easily translate the Cold Hands, Warm Heart Tea Blend (page 37) into a tincture. That way, you can take it along with you and have it on hand when you need to warm up.

2 tablespoons hawthorn tincture	1 tablespoon thyme tincture
2 tablespoons ginkgo tincture	1 tablespoon ginger tincture
2 tablespoons chamomile tincture	

1. In a measuring cup, combine the hawthorn, ginkgo, chamomile, thyme, and ginger tinctures.

2. Transfer the mixture into a 4-ounce dropper bottle.

3. Label and date the tincture blend.

4. Take 1 to 2 dropperfuls (25 to 50 drops) in 1 to 2 ounces of water or juice 2 or 3 times a day.

5. Store the tincture blend in a cool, dark place, where it will last for several years.

> **Tip:** Add this tincture to a hot cup of the Cold Hands, Warm Heart Tea (page 37) to amplify its healing properties!

Digestion

When I set out to write this book, I asked a lot of people how emotional upsets affect them. I was surprised to find that—almost universally—people feel it in their throat, esophagus, and gut. I should have known, since digestion has always been a problem for me and all of my loved ones! Anxiety manifests in the gut as a change in appetite, trouble swallowing, slower or faster digestion, and constipation or diarrhea.

That's a lot to unpack, right? Well, gut issues can mostly be addressed by simply soothing and calming the smooth muscle and nerves that make up the majority of your digestive tract. You can encourage good digestion by providing hydration, bulk, and fiber. And if your stomach is too upset to tolerate food, perhaps a smoothie will go down. Bitters may also help.

Digestivi-Tea Blend
15 (1-CUP) SERVINGS

This tea is tasty and eases many symptoms of poor digestion, such as cramps, bloating, indigestion, and nausea. Some people have trouble swallowing when they're really struggling emotionally. A little liquid can help get the action started, but it's even better to drink a nice hot tea with herbs specifically blended for nervous digestion.

¼ cup catnip	¼ cup lemon balm
¼ cup chopped ginger root	

1. In a large bowl, combine the catnip, ginger, and lemon balm.

2. Transfer the tea blend to an airtight container. Label and date the blend.

3. To use, add 1 rounded teaspoon to an infuser and place in a 10-ounce mug.

4. Cover with just-boiled water and steep for 5 to 7 minutes. Remove the infuser.

5. This is particularly good after meals. Drink up to 3 times a day.

6. Store in a cool, dry place out of direct sunlight. This will keep for a year.

Nervous Tummy Tincture
MAKES 4 OUNCES

In our family, we call it "feeling urp-y." You know, there's too much acid and gas, and everything either sits in the gut for a long time (making you feel miserable) or flies through your intestines (resulting in flatulence). Turn to this handy tincture when you need to calm and soothe your digestive tract.

3 tablespoons thyme tincture

3 tablespoons chamomile tincture

2 tablespoons spearmint tincture

1. In a measuring cup, combine the thyme, chamomile, and spearmint tinctures.

2. Transfer the mixture into a 4-ounce dropper bottle.

3. Label and date the tincture blend.

4. Take 1 to 2 dropperfuls (25 to 50 drops) added to herbal, green, or weak black tea 2 to 3 times a day.

5. Store the tincture blend in a cool, dark place, where it will last for several years.

Smoothie for Indigestion and GERD
MAKES 2 (8- TO 10-OUNCE) SMOOTHIES

It is miserable to deal with indigestion or GERD on a daily (or nightly) basis. I had a hard time with it for years and even took medication for a while. It's very important not to continually expose the esophagus to stomach acid. I found that if I felt bloated after a meal, it would eventually become painful. Eating some kind of raw fruit or vegetable an hour or so before bed seemed to really help, and carrots were my go-to. Years later, I learned that carrots are advised for these conditions in Ayurvedic medicine! This smoothie makes a great meal, especially breakfast.

½ cup chopped carrots

½ cup pineapple chunks

½ cup oat milk

1 large banana

¼ cup fresh spearmint

¼ cup fresh plantain

1 tablespoon marshmallow root powder

1 tablespoon fresh ginger

¼ teaspoon fresh or dried thyme

4 or 5 ice cubes

CONTINUES →

1. In a blender, combine the carrots, pineapple, oat milk, banana, spearmint, plantain, marshmallow root powder, ginger, thyme, and ice cubes.

2. Blend for a few minutes until the greens are well incorporated and the mixture is liquefied.

3. Store any leftover smoothie in the refrigerator and use within 2 days.

> **Tip:** Sipping a few ounces of this smoothie an hour before bed can settle the stomach.

Digestive Bitters
MAKES 2 OUNCES

Bitter taste stimulates the digestive system and prepares it to receive and digest food. It signals salivation to start, stomach acid to be produced, and bile to get ready to start working. They're bitter—no two ways about it—and you need to taste the bitterness for it to work. There are a lot of bitters on the market, or you can make your own. Nearly everyone can benefit from taking bitters 15 minutes before meals.

1 tablespoon blue vervain tincture

1 tablespoon motherwort tincture

1 tablespoon chamomile tincture

1 tablespoon ginger tincture

1. In a measuring cup, combine the blue vervain, chamomile, motherwort, and ginger tinctures.

2. Transfer the mixture into a 2-ounce dropper bottle.

3. Label and date the tincture blend.

4. Add 15 to 25 drops to an ounce of water and drink it 15 minutes before a meal.

5. Store the bitters in a cool, dark place, where it will last for several years.

> **Tip:** Make sure you taste the bitters. That doesn't mean that they must be savored, but don't disguise the flavor.

Focus

Swimming through muddy water, walking through heavy fog, feeling like you're not completely awake—that lack of focus is exhausting, and sometimes a cup or two of coffee doesn't cut through it. You don't need a severe case of ADD to look to herbs for help. In the recipes that follow, you'll find those that support brain function and improve your energy level.

Foundational Focus Elixir
MAKES ABOUT 3 OUNCES

This combination is specifically helpful for those periods of time when you have to pull out the stops for a week or two. Things like cramming for finals, writing a term paper, the last month before the house sale finally goes through, or filing taxes are examples that come to mind. It can also be useful on vacation because even though trips are something we've looked forward to all year, we push our bodies and take in so much information that a little focus can help a lot.

2 tablespoons ashwagandha

2 tablespoons rhodiola

2 tablespoons eleuthero root

2 tablespoons honey

Alcohol of choice to cover (a little more than 4 tablespoons)

1. In a small (at least 4-ounce) jar, combine the ashwagandha, rhodiola, and eleuthero.

2. Add the honey, using a knife or chopstick to combine it with the herbs.

3. Fill the rest of the jar with your alcohol of choice. Cover the jar and shake well.

4. Infuse the elixir for 2 to 4 weeks, storing it in a cool, dark place and shaking occasionally.

5. Once it's done infusing, strain the elixir and transfer it to a cropper bottle.

6. Label and date the elixir.

7. Take up to 1 teaspoon of elixir 2 times a day.

8. Store the elixir in a cool, dark place, where it will last for several years.

Tip: Avoid taking after dinner because it may make it harder to fall asleep!

Clear Thoughts Tea Blend

30 (1-CUP) SERVINGS

All the herbs and roots combined in this delicious tea work together to awaken and energize your mind. It can put a little spring in your step, too. Make this in two parts because the roots require a different extraction method than the herbal infusion.

For the syrup

1 tablespoon freshly grated ginger

1 tablespoon rhodiola

6 ounces water

⅓ cup honey

For the tea blend and the infusion

¼ cup rosemary

¼ cup astragalus

¼ cup peppermint

To make the syrup

1. In a saucepan over medium-high heat, put the ginger, the rhodiola, and water. Simmer until the mixture is reduced by half (3 ounces), about 20 minutes.

2. Strain the decoction into a bowl. Add the honey and mix well to combine.

3. Transfer the syrup to a bottle.

4. Label and date the syrup.

5. Refrigerate the syrup for up to 3 months.

To make the tea blend and the infusion

1. In a large bowl, combine the rosemary, astragalus, and peppermint.

CONTINUES →

2. Transfer the tea blend to an airtight container. Label and date the blend.

3. To use, add 1 rounded teaspoon to an infuser and place in a 10-ounce mug.

4. Cover with just-boiled water and steep for 5 minutes. Remove the infuser.

5. Add 2 teaspoons of the ginger-rhodiola syrup.

6. Store the tea blend in a cool, dry place out of direct sunlight. This will keep for a year.

Tip: The syrup can be replaced by 15 to 20 drops each of ginger and rhodiola tinctures.

Panic and Phobias

The first time I flew commercially, I didn't expect to have any qualms, because as a kid, I had many experiences flying in small four- or six-seat planes. So it came as a complete surprise that I was barely able to board. (Thankfully, a relative slipped me half of an antianxiety pill.) There are so many situations that can bring about panic: heights, enclosed spaces, various insects, public speaking, and in the worst cases, leaving the house.

It starts with perspiration, increased respiration, heart pounding, and an overwhelming desire to flee. Your knees may knock, your mouth may get dry, and you may fumble and forget important details... Depending on the situation, you'll either want to calm and slow your responses, or sharpen your wit so you can balance out your fear.

Fear of Flying Tincture
MAKES 2 OUNCES

Mild to moderate phobias, like flying, public speaking, and heights, can't always be avoided. Or if you do avoid them, doing so puts a serious dent in your full enjoyment of life. I developed this because formula because flying used to be terrifying for me. This takes the edge off and relaxes you enough that you can nod off for the flight.

2 tablespoons California poppy tincture

1 tablespoon valerian tincture

1 tablespoon ginger tincture

1. In a measuring cup, combine the California poppy, valerian, and ginger tinctures.

2. Transfer the mixture into a 2-ounce dropper bottle.

3. Label and date the tincture blend.

4. Take 1 to 2 dropperfuls (25 to 50 drops) in 1 to 2 ounces of water or juice 30 minutes before the event that causes your phobia to kick in. Repeat the dose 30 minutes later if needed.

5. Store the tincture blend in a cool, dark place, where it will last for several years.

> **Tip:** This tincture blend may make you very drowsy (which is by design for flying), but keep that in mind when taking it for other situations in which you may need to be more alert.

The Big-Day Tincture
MAKES 2 OUNCES

———————

This combo is handy for the day of a big test, a job interview, or when you're meeting someone important for the first time. Anytime a little extra brainpower is desired, give this blend a try.

2 tablespoons eleuthero tincture	½ tablespoon rhodiola tincture
1 tablespoon ashwagandha tincture	½ tablespoon ginkgo tincture

1. In a measuring cup, combine the eleuthero, ashwagandha, rhodiola, and ginkgo tinctures.

2. Transfer the mixture into a 2-ounce dropper bottle.

3. Label and date the tincture blend.

4. Take 1 to 2 dropperfuls (25 to 50 drops) in 1 to 2 ounces of water or juice shortly before the big event.

5. Store the tincture blend in a cool, dark place, where it will last for several years.

Moodiness, Cramps, or PMS

Everyone at some point knows how it feels to be bloated, wired, a little bummed out, and kind of queasy, right? We always think of those symptoms as women's issues, but they can happen to everyone. The herbal remedies that follow are intended for anyone who is cranky no matter their gender or age.

Balance Tea Blend
50 (1-CUP) SERVINGS

———————

I've blended this lovely tea to address some of the most annoying aspects of premenstrual syndrome, but please don't keep it hidden and only pull it out a few days each month. Instead, serve it anytime your spirit is flagging and causing physical symptoms. Next to each ingredient you'll find the reason it went into the blend to help explain its usefulness.

½ cup nettle (diuretic and supports the adrenals)	¼ cup mimosa bark (lifts mood)
½ cup lemon balm (calms nerves)	1 tablespoon ginger powder (soothes tummy and pain)
¼ cup catnip (calms nerves and tummy)	Honey (optional)
	Lemon (optional)

1. In a large bowl, combine the nettle, lemon balm, catnip, mimosa bark, and ginger powder.

CONTINUES →

2. Transfer the tea blend to an airtight container. Label and date the blend.

3. To use, add 1 rounded teaspoon to an infuser and place in a 10-ounce mug.

4. Cover with just-boiled water and steep for 5 to 7 minutes. Remove the infuser.

5. Sweeten with honey and lemon (if using).

6. Store the tea blend in a cool, dry place out of direct sunlight. This will keep for a year.

> **Tip:** Take your time to relax and drink this tea slowly; put your feet up to help fluids move.

Monday Mornings Tincture
MAKES 2 OUNCES

The herbs in this blend address mood swings, emotional balance, and aches and pains. It's too bitter to drink as a tea, but the tincture can be used to encourage digestion in addition to lifting a blue mood.

2 tablespoons motherwort tincture

1 tablespoon lemon balm tincture

1 tablespoon blue vervain tincture

1. In a measuring cup, combine the motherwort, lemon balm, and blue vervain tinctures.

2. Transfer the mixture into a 2-ounce dropper bottle.

3. Label and date the tincture blend.

4. Take 25 to 40 drops in 1 ounce of water or juice and drink quickly (remember: it's bitter!) up to 2 times a day.

5. Store the tincture blend in a cool, dark place, where it will last for several years.

Herbal Hot Pad
MAKES 1 PAD

There are several of these hot pads in my home, and there's nothing like a warm, fragrant weight on the lower belly to soothe cramps. They are useful for so many things—such as strained muscles, gas pains, and cold feet—that you may find that one is not enough.

2 cups rice

½ cup lavender

½ cup peppermint

1 knee-high sports sock

1. In a medium bowl, combine the rice, lavender, and peppermint.

2. Carefully fill the sock with the rice and herb mixture.

3. Secure the open end of the sock by either sewing it shut or tying it in a knot.

4. Place the hot pad into the microwave and heat for 30 to 60 seconds.

5. If it is too hot, place a towel between the hot pad and your body until it cools sufficiently.

6. This hot pad can be used over and over. It can also go into the freezer to be used as a cold pack; put it into a plastic bag first to avoid moisture buildup.

Tip: As an alternative to using a sock, you can sew a 4-by-12-inch tube with a tight weave fabric (I like cotton). After filling the fabric tube with the rice and herb mixture, you'll need to sew the open end shut.

Recovering from the Storm

When upsetting things happen, they pass, and we are left with all this leftover adrenaline. We feel worked up and depleted at the same time. Tense and exhausted—"wired and tired"—all at once. These remedies may be just what we need.

Pick-Me-Up Tea Blend
25 (1-CUP) SERVINGS

This is a good tea to drink when it isn't easy to toss off the tense energy of an event that shook you off-balance. Perhaps you still have work to do and people to see. It would be so much easier to blow everything off, but there's no way around it; the show must go on. Taking a moment to sip and breathe deeply will make all the difference.

2 tablespoons ashwagandha

2 tablespoons mimosa bark

¼ cup lemon balm

¼ cup holy basil

2 tablespoons peppermint

Honey (optional)

1. In a large bowl, combine the ashwagandha, mimosa bark, lemon balm, holy basil, and peppermint.

2. Transfer the tea blend to an airtight container. Label and date the blend.

3. To use, add 1½ teaspoons to an infuser and place in a 10-ounce mug.

4. Cover with just-boiled water and steep for 7 to 10 minutes. Remove the infuser.

5. Sweeten with honey (if using) and drink slowly.

6. Store in a cool, dry place out of direct sunlight. This will keep for a year.

Tip: While drinking this tea, stay in the moment—not before, not ahead, just now. The time spent and the tea can help you reconsolidate all of your tattered bits and come back to a place of calm.

Anxiety-Interrupted Tincture
MAKES 1 OUNCE

My cat was a stray, and after she chose this house, there was no way she was going to let any other dog, cat, bird, rabbit, or squirrel usurp her. Many years later, she still gets worked up when she senses an intruder. It takes her a while to stop growling and fretting. That feeling happens to us, too, and that's when we can use a dose of this tincture. As humans, we can find ourselves in situations that make us feel defensive. It takes some time to get over the feeling, but this blend helps shrink that time so we can get on with our days.

2 teaspoons holy basil tincture

2 teaspoons hawthorn tincture

2 teaspoons lemon balm tincture

1. In a measuring cup, combine the holy basil, lemon balm, and hawthorn tinctures.

2. Transfer the mixture into a 1-ounce dropper bottle.

3. Label and date the tincture blend.

4. Take 1 dropperful (25 to 30 drops) in 1 ounce of water or juice as needed along with a couple of relaxing breaths.

5. Store the tincture blend in a cool, dark place, where it will last for several years.

Unwind Syrup
MAKES 8 OUNCES

I find this blend to be so comforting and versatile that it's become a go-to in our house. Not only are the herbs relaxing and calming, they also improve digestion. This is just the thing you need when it's hard to leave behind work or school worries. Keeping it available as syrup means that a teaspoon or three can be added to teas or served over ice cream, oatmeal, or pieces of cut fresh fruit.

½ cup mint

½ cup chamomile

2 tablespoons lavender

½ cup honey

1. In a small saucepan with a lid, combine the mint, chamomile, and lavender. Set aside.

2. In a separate pan, heat enough boiling water to just cover the herb mixture. Add the water to the saucepan with the herbs, cover, and steep for 4 to 8 hours or overnight.

3. Strain the mixture. Heat the strained tea to a simmer.

4. Measure out ½ cup of the liquid. If there is less than ½ cup, add very hot water to make up the difference. If there is more than ½ cup, either simmer to reduce or discard the excess.

5. Add the honey to the saucepan and mix well to combine.

6. Cool the syrup and transfer it to an 8-ounce bottle.

7. Label and date the syrup.

8. Store in the refrigerator and use within 9 months.

> **Tip:** If you'd prefer to make this syrup with sugar rather than honey, you can! Simply add ¾ cup of sugar to the ½ cup of liquid and bring the mixture to a boil for 3 minutes. Follow the same instructions from step 6 on.

Sleep Issues

Sleep problems are as universal as issues with digestion. There are a lot of ways to encourage sleep. For instance, keep the bedroom for only sleep and lovemaking. Stick to a schedule, and avoid daytime naps (my personal downfall). Don't eat for several hours before bed. Turn off screens at least 30 minutes before bed, and instead read or listen to relaxing music. When we get to depression, we'll talk about sleeping too much.

Go to Sleep Now Tincture
MAKES 4 OUNCES

Sleep makes such a difference in how well we can manage in the world, but so often it's elusive when we need it the most. Sleep resets our brains and puts us back together. I love this tincture because it is a relaxing sedative and slows a racing brain to a crawl.

4 tablespoons California poppy tincture

2 tablespoons passionflower tincture

2 tablespoons skullcap tincture

1. In a measuring cup, combine the California poppy, passionflower, and skullcap tinctures.

2. Transfer the mixture into a 4-ounce dropper bottle.

3. Label and date the tincture blend.

4. Take 1 to 2 dropperfuls (30 to 50 drops) 30 minutes before bed.

5. Store the tincture blend in a cool, dark place, where it will last for several years.

> **Tip:** Imagine there's a blackboard (or maybe a whiteboard?) inside your head or behind your eyelids. Every time you become aware of a thought, slowly envision an eraser wiping it away.

Lavender Stuffed Animal
MAKES 1 STUFFED ANIMAL

Years ago, I had to spend a week in the hospital, and my husband wasn't able to take much time off work to be with me. Overnights alone in the hospital were the worst, and I'd

CONTINUES →

cry myself to sleep. On day three, he showed up with a teddy bear. It may sound silly, but I clung to that thing like a life raft. It's a comforting and effective sleep aid for when anxiety makes it hard to fall asleep and remain there.

3-by-5-inch muslin bag

¾ cup lavender

1 inexpensive medium-size stuffed animal

1. Fill the muslin bag with lavender and sew the open end shut.

2. Using a seam ripper, open a seam about 4 inches long somewhere along the side or chest of the stuffed animal.

3. Remove some of the stuffing to make room for the lavender-filled muslin bag.

4. Place the bag of lavender inside the stuffed animal.

5. Carefully sew the stuffed animal shut again.

6. Give the stuffed animal a hug. (See what I mean?)

Restless Circular Thinking Tincture
MAKES 2 OUNCES

Circular thinking is pretty common with anxiety. We're talking about it here under sleep, but it can also manifest as someone working through a problem, talking it through, and then starting all over in the beginning. Over and over again.

2 tablespoons passionflower tincture

½ tablespoon lavender tincture

1½ tablespoons valerian tincture

1. In a measuring cup, combine the passionflower, valerian, and lavender tinctures.

2. Transfer the mixture into a 4-ounce dropper bottle.

3. Label and date the tincture blend.

4. Take 1 dropperful (20 to 30 drops) in 1 ounce of water or juice. Repeat the dose 30 minutes later if needed. This can be used up to 3 times a day.

5. Store the tincture blend in a cool, dark place, where it will last for several years.

Tip: This recipe can also be made into a tea by following the same proportions.

System Support

No matter what we learn about working with symptoms once they show up, it's far better to be strong and grounded to meet problems head-on. Anxiety wreaks havoc on so many organs that it takes a toll on the immune system. That needs to be supported and strengthened. Try to include some of these immune-stimulating herbs every day, especially when the days are shorter in the winter months.

Build-Me-Up Tea Blend
35 (1-CUP) SERVINGS

This tea is a great strengthener that at the same time can make it easier to face things we'd prefer not to face.

¼ cup echinacea (aerial parts)

¼ cup eleuthero root

½ cup elderberries

¼ cup astragalus

¼ cup thyme

Honey (optional)

Lemon (optional)

1. In a large bowl, combine the echinacea, eleuthero, elderberries, astragalus, and thyme.

2. Transfer the tea blend to an airtight container. Label and date the blend.

3. To use, add 1 rounded teaspoon to an infuser and place in a 10-ounce mug.

4. Cover with just-boiled water and steep for 5 to 7 minutes. Remove the infuser.

5. Sweeten with honey and lemon (if using).

6. Store in a cool, dry place out of direct sunlight. This will keep for a year.

Strengthening Tonic
MAKES 1 QUART

This is an elixir, but we're calling it a tonic because its entire purpose is to build up and "tonify" your immune system! You'll want to make a large amount so you can take it daily, especially over the winter. The sweetness of the remedy makes it a welcome one for even children. All the ingredients come together to boost your immune system while protecting and strengthening your nervous system.

½ cup nettle

¼ cup elderberries

¼ cup astragalus

¼ cup skullcap

¼ cup St. John's wort

¼ cup eleuthero root

1 tablespoon rosemary

1½ cups honey

2½ cups alcohol of choice (some will be absorbed by the dry herbs)

1. To a large-mouth, 48-ounce jar, put the nettle, elderberries, astragalus, skullcap, St. John's wort, eleuthero, and rosemary.

2. Add the honey and use a long spoon to combine it with the herbs.

3. Add the alcohol and stir until the honey is mostly incorporated with the alcohol.

4. Cover the jar and shake well.

5. Infuse the tonic for 2 to 4 weeks, storing it in a cool, dark place and shaking daily.

6. Once it's done infusing, strain the tonic and transfer it to smaller bottles.

7. Label and date the bottles.

8. Take 1 teaspoon each morning to start the day.

CONTINUES →

9. The tonic will keep for a year at room temperature

> **Tip:** The elixir will separate while it's infusing, and that's normal—hence the need to shake it daily.

Comforting Immunity Stew
4 SERVINGS

Yep, this is a meal. Many of the herbs that are discussed in these pages can also be included in the kitchen. The more we become familiar with them and let them assist us in the ways our ancestors did, the better off we'll be. This stew can be altered in a lot of ways, and ingredients like oatmeal or medicinal mushrooms make terrific additions. Even the cayenne, onion, and garlic in the recipe provide wonderful support for the immune system. If you can find burdock root, typically called *gobo* in Asian markets, by all means, add that, too!

1 onion, chopped

3 cloves garlic, minced

1 tablespoon minced fresh ginger root

1 tablespoon coconut or olive oil

8 ounces sliced mushrooms

1 quart broth (chicken or vegetable)

½ cup carrot slices

½ cup celery slices

5 or 6 astragalus slices

1 tablespoon thyme

1 teaspoon cayenne pepper

1 cup chopped fresh or ¼ cup dry nettle

1. In a skillet over medium-high heat, sauté the onion, garlic, and ginger in coconut oil for 5 minutes until soft.

2. Add the mushrooms and continue to sauté for 3 minutes. Remove the skillet from the heat and set aside.

3. In a medium stockpot, heat the broth and add the carrots, celery, and astragalus.

4. Add the reserved sautéed onion mixture to the stockpot.

5. If you would prefer the stew to be a little more soupy, add some water. Bring the stew to a boil.

6. Reduce to a low simmer for 15 minutes.

7. Add the thyme, cayenne pepper, and nettle and simmer for 3 more minutes.

8. Remove and discard the astragalus slices.

9. Serve with some crusty bread.

> **Tip:** You can add other veggies (or even some protein) if you like. Cooked beans or lentils (½ cup) are very good.

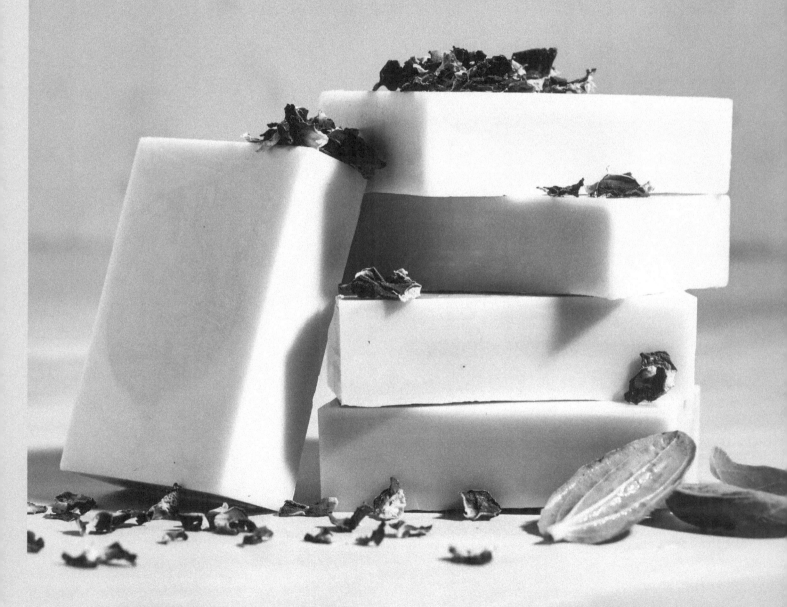

SOFT SKIN
LOTION BAR
Page 57

CHAPTER 5

Depression

As with most emotional conditions, depression presents in a spectrum of intensity. Mild depression may look like a lack of interest in a hobby or socializing, while severe depression can keep you in bed for days, unable to shower or get dressed. And there are many stages in between. Most people have experienced depression at some point in their lives. Perhaps it comes with increasing feelings of low self-esteem, a mood that some sufferers call "the black dog," a lack of concentration and energy, mixed-up sleep patterns, or a change in appetite.

Depression can be caused by specific events—or it may arrive for no reason at all. Attention to nutrition (including possible food allergies and sensitivities), exercise, sleep, and exposure to natural light can help keep us on an even keel, but sometimes depression shows up out of the blue anyway.

When my daughter moved across the country, it hit me hard. She'd gone away from home to go to college, but now, we'd no longer have holidays or summers. This was real.

I thought I was dealing with it, but I went to the doctor about something else, and she asked me to fill out a questionnaire. It was a series of questions with answers ranging from "never" to "always." It was meant to measure depression, which I didn't think was the issue. When I was finished and looked at the answers, it was clear that it was indeed the issue, and whatever took me in to see the doctor was actually a symptom of depression. I started walking every day, eating whole foods, and working with some herbs, promising that if I started feeling worse, we'd discuss it. Being aware of it helped me get a handle on it.

Depression can be insidious and overpowering. Please don't ever feel as if you have to go through it alone. It isn't anything to be ashamed of or to hide from or to "fix" because otherwise we are "broken." We don't do that with other things that cause pain. I'll never understand how we've come to believe that we have to keep these things to ourselves. I've often thought that just as we get our teeth cleaned twice a year, we should have mental health checkups twice a year.

Common symptoms of depression include apathy, general discontent, guilt, hopelessness, loss of interest (or pleasure) in activities, mood swings, sadness, agitation, crying, irritability, avoiding social situations, sleeping too much (or too little), eating too much (or too little), and inability to concentrate.

Body Care for Self-Esteem

It's really hard to get out of that sloppy (possibly dirty) T-shirt and get cleaned up some days. The irony is that very often the acts of taking a shower, putting on clean clothes, changing the sheets, and opening the curtains can all bring an immediate mood improvement. Add some pampering, and although it may be temporary, we feel better. Feeling grungy is part of a cycle in which we can't leave the house because we need a shower, and we can't get a shower because we don't feel like bothering, and around and around we go! Some of the following preparations may help.

After-Shower Oil Spray
3 TO 4 (½-CUP) APPLICATIONS

In depression, grooming is often one of the first things to go. The herbs used in this oil spray have antibiotic and antibacterial properties and offer some deodorizing properties. Especially in cold weather or with older skin, a light spray of oil after the shower makes you feel more comfortable in your skin and keeps dry skin itches from getting a foothold.

¼ cup witch hazel

2 tablespoons sage-infused olive oil

2 tablespoons thyme-infused olive oil

2 tablespoons peppermint-infused olive oil

2 tablespoons lavender-infused olive oil

1. In a measuring cup, combine the witch hazel and the: sage-, peppermint-, thyme-, and lavender-infused olive oils.

2. Using a small funnel, transfer the oil mixture into a spray bottle.

3. After a bath or shower, spray the oil mixture onto barely dry skin to soften and moisturize the body.

4. Massage the oil in well.

5. Make in small batches so it remains fresh and use within 1 month.

6. This will separate, so shake well before each use.

Bright Eyes Compress
ENOUGH FOR 1 APPLICATION

Disturbed sleep, too much screen time, and crying can make your eyes feel sore, tired, and swollen. Just 15 minutes with one of these will help your eyes feel brighter and look better. It may even improve your overall outlook.

2 tea bags (mint, chamomile, or echinacea)

1. Brew a strong cup of tea using your choice of tea bags.

2. Cool the tea bags and place one on each eye. Rest them there for 15 minutes or so.

3. Meanwhile, relax and meditate or listen to soothing or upbeat music.

4. If you fall asleep, the tea bags won't hurt anything if they fall off.

5. Discard or compost the tea bags when you are through with them.

Tip: If you can't get your hands on tea bags, cotton balls saturated with cool water also work in a pinch.

Dry Shampoo
5 TO 10 APPLICATIONS (DEPENDING ON HAIR LENGTH)

You just have to leave the house for a couple hours to run errands, but the effort of a shower, getting dressed, driving . . . it's all too much. Dry shampoo can freshen the appearance of hair enough to pull off not showering for a little while longer. The measurements in this recipe are flexible. If your hair is dark, use more powdered herbs and less arrowroot or powder.

¼ cup arrowroot (or any kind of body powder)

1 heaping tablespoon powdered mint

1 heaping tablespoon powdered lavender

1. In a measuring cup, combine the arrowroot, mint, and lavender. Mix the ingredients very well and transfer into a small jar, ideally with a shaker top.

CONTINUES →

2. Place a scant teaspoon of the mixture in the palm of one hand and distribute over both palms.

3. Lightly massage it into the hair, particularly near the scalp. It will absorb excess oil and give the hair volume.

4. Brush thoroughly.

5. Wash your hair before going to bed because the dry shampoo will weigh the hair down and may leave it feeling gunky the next day.

Tip: I save every jar with a shaker top (spices, Parmesan cheese, etc.) for just this kind of thing.

Rejuvenating Facial Mask
MAKES ENOUGH FOR 1 FACIAL MASK

This basic recipe allows for substitutions depending on your skin type and the herbs at your disposal. For dry to normal skin, use any blend of nettle, mint, lemon balm, marshmallow powder, or rose to make up your ½ cup of dry herbs. For oily skin, use any blend of sage, mint, nettle, or lavender.

½ cup dry herbs

½ medium cucumber, peeled and seeded

2 tablespoons witch hazel

1. In a blender, add your custom herb blend, the cucumber, and the witch hazel.

2. Blend until it forms a fairly uniform paste.

3. Apply a thick layer to your face and relax for 15 minutes. Rinse with warm water and lightly pat dry.

Tip: No cucumber? Try using half an apple or a handful of berries.

Shine On Hair Rinse
MAKES 3 APPLICATIONS

Depression feels dull. Personally, when I'm down, it seems like the intensity of my senses has been turned way down—a lot like when I have a bad cold. It is always surprising how much better everything feels when I'm cleaned up and presentable. This rinse is a simple bit of self-care that restores shine by smoothing down the outer surface of the hair.

½ cup rosemary

½ cup lavender

1 quart water

2 cups apple cider vinegar

1. In a heatproof bowl or wide-mouth quart jar, combine the rosemary and lavender.

2. Boil the water and pour over the herb mixture. Steep for an hour.

3. Strain the mixture and combine the remaining liquid with the apple cider vinegar.

4. After washing your hair, apply 2 cups of the hair rinse. Rinse out with fresh water.

5. Store the remaining hair rinse in an air-tight container and use within a month.

Soft Skin Lotion Bar
2 (1¼-OUNCE) BARS

This is a form of a balm or salve, but the beeswax content is increased so that it is a solid. It's ideal for rougher spots on the body, such as elbows and heels, but also feels wonderful applied on your hands. I like to rub this on my feet and then immediately put on fluffy socks before climbing into bed. I've also used it with socks on my hands when they're really dry.

1½ tablespoons rose-infused olive oil	1½ tablespoons beeswax pastilles
1½ tablespoons plantain-infused olive oil	Ice cube tray (silicone trays work really well, but plastic ones are okay, too)

1. In a measuring cup, add the rose-infused olive oil, plantain-infused olive oil, and beeswax. Combine well and then melt in the microwave in 30-second increments.

2. When the beeswax starts to soften, stir the mixture well with a chopstick before additional heating. (The wax will continue to melt into the oil while being stirred.)

3. Once all the beeswax is melted, pour the lotion mixture into two or three cavities of an ice cube tray.

4. Freeze for 30 to 60 minutes.

5. Smack the ice cube tray sharply on the counter to dislodge from the lotion cubes.

6. Store the lotion cubes in an airtight container to keep them clean. Use within 6 months.

Tip: See page 25 for instructions for how to infuse herbs into oil.

Stimulating Astringent
MAKES 1 CUP

A nice, invigorating astringent brightens up your face and may temporarily bring you out from under a dark cloud.

1 cup witch hazel	2 tablespoons holy basil
2 tablespoons chamomile	2 tablespoons peppermint
2 tablespoons rose	2 tablespoons apple cider vinegar

1. In a small jar, add the witch hazel, chamomile, rose, holy basil, and peppermint. Infuse the mixture for 2 weeks.

2. Strain the witch hazel and discard the herbs, pressing out as much of the liquid as possible.

CONTINUES →

3. Combine the witch hazel mixture and the apple cider vinegar and pour it into an 8-ounce bottle.

4. Apply to the face and neck using cotton balls no more than 1 or 2 times a day.

5. The astringent should keep indefinitely.

Concentration

Having a "who cares" kind of day? Part of that might be coming from an inability to concentrate. Whether it comes from a lack of interest or an inability doesn't matter too much when you're in the thick of it. For most of us, the ability to function and process information is critical, and a few hours—or, at most, a couple of days—off is all we can afford to lose.

I find that choosing a small task that can be completed and feels like an accomplishment can help get me back on track—simple tasks such as putting away folded laundry, cleaning the bathroom sink, or going through the stack of junk mail on the dining room table to clear a space. Clear surfaces are very helpful for me. My daughter fine-tunes her budget. My sister files paperwork. We all have tasks we can do without much critical thinking that help reset our ability to "think straight."

Spicy Concentration Brew
8 (1-CUP) SERVINGS

It's important to take time out and recognize that something is going on because you can't work on something that hasn't been acknowledged. While drinking this Spicy Concentration Brew, plan and mentally run through a task that might help you feel more focused. I mentally practice something several times before starting.

2 tablespoons ashwagandha	8 fresh ginger root slices
2 tablespoons holy basil	

1. In a small bowl, combine the ashwagandha and holy basil.

2. Transfer the tea blend to an airtight container. Label and date the blend.

3. To use, put 1 slice of fresh ginger in the bottom of a 10-ounce mug along with an infuser holding 1 rounded teaspoon of the herb blend.

4. Cover with just-boiled water and steep for 3 to 5 minutes. Remove the infuser.

5. Drink up to 2 cups a day.

6. Store in a cool, dry place out of direct sunlight.

> **Tip:** I leave the ginger and herbs in the mug while drinking for some added heat!

Clari-Tea Blend
8 (1-CUP) SERVINGS

This tea is also very good for mentally preparing to begin a task or to recharge when concentration begins to flag. A lemon wedge makes a nice addition to this tea blend.

3 tablespoons rosemary	Honey (optional)
1 tablespoon ginkgo	Lemon (optional)

1. In a small bowl, combine the rosemary and ginkgo.

2. Transfer the tea blend to an airtight container. Label and date the blend.

3. To use, add 1 rounded teaspoon to an infuser and place in a 10-ounce mug.

4. Cover with just-boiled water and steep for 3 to 5 minutes. Remove the infuser.

5. Sweeten with honey and lemon (if using).

6. Drink 1 cup a day.

7. Store in a cool, dry place out of direct sunlight.

Attention Drops
MAKES 4 OUNCES

This combination may at first seem counterproductive because we think of some of the herbs as being very relaxing, but it helps quiet the depressing or anxious thoughts that steal attentiveness while increasing mental energy and supporting a healthy thought processes.

2 tablespoons catnip tincture	1 tablespoon chamomile tincture
2 tablespoons ashwagandha tincture	1 tablespoon lemon balm tincture
1 tablespoon rhodiola tincture	1 tablespoon milky oats tincture

1. In a measuring cup, combine the catnip, ashwagandha, rhodiola, chamomile, lemon balm, and milky oats tinctures.

2. Transfer the mixture into a 4-ounce dropper bottle.

3. Label and date the tincture blend.

4. Take 1 dropperful (25 to 30 drops) in 1 ounce of water or juice. Repeat the dose 30 minutes later if needed. Can be used up to 3 times a day.

5. Store the tincture blend in a cool, dark place, where it will last for several years.

Agitation Cessation Blend
MAKES 4 OUNCES

You don't often associate agitation with depression—and yet it can be a symptom. Agitation might show up as pacing the floor, biting nails, twisting hair, cracking knuckles, or any activity that is a release. Unfortunately, these are not

CONTINUES →

particularly productive ways to channel that energy. If they become a means of self-harm, please talk to a professional. This tincture can help quell any swirling, out-of-control feelings.

2 tablespoons skullcap tincture

2 tablespoons catnip tincture

2 tablespoons St. John's wort tincture

2 tablespoons passionflower tincture

1. In a measuring cup, combine the skull-cap, St. John's wort, catnip, and passion-flower tinctures.

2. Transfer the mixture into a 4-ounce dropper bottle.

3. Label and date the tincture blend.

4. Take 1 dropperful (25 to 30 drops) in 1 to 2 ounces of water or juice up to 4 times a day.

5. Store the tincture blend in a cool, dark place, where it will last for several years.

Moody Blues

Everybody gets the blues sometimes. They don't even need a reason to show up. My grandmother used to say that she was feeling low. This is generally a very mild and temporary form of depression, and there are lots of ways to usher that dark cloud on its way. Get out with a friend, turn up some music and sing or dance along—or whip up a potion!

Baby Blues Tea Blend
35 TO 40 (1-CUP) SERVINGS

Sadly, in our society, postpartum depression is minimized in much the same way menstrual cramps are minimized. We allow moms to question themselves and suffer needlessly. If you are a new mom, try to get sleep when you can, get enough to eat, accept *any* help that is offered, and ask for help if you need it! Herbs really love mothers. Mix this blend up before your due date, and it will be ready for you if you need it.

½ cup holy basil

¼ cup oatstraw

¼ cup catnip

2 tablespoons blue vervain

2 tablespoons skullcap

1. In a medium bowl, combine the holy basil, oatstraw, catnip, blue vervain, and skullcap.

2. Transfer the tea blend to an airtight container. Label and date the blend.

3. To use, add 1 rounded teaspoon to an infuser and place in a 10-ounce mug.

4. Cover with just-boiled water and steep for 5 to 7 minutes. Remove the infuser.

5. Drink up to 3 times a day.

6. Store in a cool, dry place out of direct sunlight. This will keep for a year.

> **Tip:** The herbs in this blend are considered safe for nursing mothers. If the mother is not nursing, ashwagandha and St. John's wort make good additions.

Back to Center Tincture

MAKES 3 OUNCES

Depression can make us feel like a ship that has no anchor, being buffeted and thrown about by the whims of the weather and currents of the water. Running aground or crashing into rocks seems to be almost expected. The following blend can help us return to our center and drop that anchor to ground ourselves.

2 tablespoons milky oats tincture

2 tablespoons ashwagandha tincture

2 tablespoons rose tincture

1. In a measuring cup, combine the milky oats, ashwagandha, and rose tinctures.

2. Transfer the mixture into a small dropper bottle.

3. Label and date the tincture blend.

4. Take 25 to 40 drops in 1 to 2 ounces of water up to 3 times a day.

5. Store in a cool, dark place, where it will last for several years.

Daily Mood Support Honey

MAKES ABOUT 1 CUP

This honey can be used to sweeten any tea, morning oatmeal, or cereal or enjoyed by the teaspoon. Add a little to some vinegar and use it as a salad dressing. There are lots of ways to get a little daily mood support.

2 tablespoons ashwagandha

2 tablespoons holy basil

2 tablespoons rhodiola

2 tablespoons eleuthero root

1 cup raw honey

1. In a pint jar, combine the ashwagandha, holy basil, rhodiola, eleuthero, and honey. (The combined herbs will amount to ½ cup.)

2. Mix well, making sure to remove all the air bubbles.

3. Seal the jar, and label and date the blend.

4. Infuse the honey for 3 to 4 weeks, storing it in a cool, dark place. The herbs will migrate to the top of the honey, so each day, turn the jar over.

5. When done infusing, pour the honey through a fine-mesh strainer, letting it strain for a few hours to get as much of the honey as possible.

6. Transfer the herbal honey into a jar. Label and date the blend.

7. Honey is very stable at room temperature, especially when stored in a cool, dark place. It will last at least a year.

Dark Cloud Vinegar Tonic
MAKES ABOUT 2 CUPS

In this preparation, we'll be using alcohol and vinegar in order to pull out all the properties in these herbs. This isn't quite a tincture and isn't quite a vinegar, but put it together and it's the ideal tonic for sad days.

¼ cup chamomile

¼ cup milky oats

¼ cup blue vervain

¼ cup mimosa

1 cup alcohol of choice

1 cup apple cider vinegar

½ cup honey

1. In a 24- to 32-ounce jar, put the chamomile, milky oats, blue vervain, mimosa, alcohol, apple cider vinegar, and honey.

2. Mix well, being certain to remove air bubbles.

3. Cover the jar opening with parchment paper, and then screw the lid on tightly.

4. Label and date the blend.

5. Infuse the tonic for at least 2 weeks, storing it in a cool, dark place and shaking daily.

6. Strain the mixture, pressing as much of the liquid as possible from the herbs.

7. Transfer the tonic to a pint jar. Label and date the blend.

8. Take 1 teaspoon (in water or juice) up to 4 times a day.

9. Store in a cool, dark place, where it will last for several years.

Seasonal Affective Disorder (SAD)

The lack of sunlight in winter affects many people, literally putting them "under the weather." Long stretches of cloudy, gloomy weather in the summer do the same thing to me, and people who don't get outside regularly are particularly vulnerable. Vitamin D supplementation is a good idea, as is getting outside and exposing as much skin as you're comfortable with to the light when it's warm enough. There are also special light bulbs that people swear by.

Liquid Sunshine Tincture
MAKES 4 OUNCES

There is no such thing as liquid sunshine, but if there were, it would likely look something like this bottle of herbal cheer. St. John's wort got its name because it blooms around the summer solstice, which coincides with the Feast of St. John on June 24. To celebrate the longest day of light, the blossoms were gathered and used to create head wreathes and bouquets. Bonfires were lit to represent the light.

2 tablespoons St. John's wort tincture

2 tablespoons lemon balm tincture

2 tablespoons mimosa tincture

2 tablespoons rhodiola tincture

1. In a measuring cup, combine the St. John's wort, mimosa, lemon balm, and rhodiola tinctures.

2. Transfer the mixture into a 4-ounce dropper bottle.

3. Label and date the tincture blend.

4. Take 1 dropperful (25 to 30 drops) in 1 ounce of water or juice up to 3 times a day as needed.

5. Store the tincture blend in a cool, dark place, where it will last for several years.

Sun in Winter Tea Blend
30 (1-CUP) SERVINGS

Take this blend along to work and drink it during the day to keep a sunny mood.

⅓ cup lemon balm

⅓ cup holy basil

⅓ cup rose

Honey (optional)

Lemon (optional)

1. In a large bowl, combine the lemon balm, holy basil, and rose.

2. Transfer the tea blend to an airtight container. Label and date the blend.

3. To use, add 1 rounded teaspoon to an infuser and place in a 10-ounce mug.

4. Cover with just-boiled water and steep for about 5 minutes. Remove the infuser

5. Sweeten with honey and lemon (if using) for even more sunshine power!

6. Enjoy liberally.

7. Store in a cool, dry place out of direct sunlight. This will keep for a year.

Tired—Get Up and Go

There are several physiological conditions that can cause chronic exhaustion, so you'll want to get anything that doesn't go away checked out. However, we live in a world that constantly wears us down. The days are too short, there's too much to do, and for whatever reason, some of us are more susceptible to trying to fulfill all the demands placed on our shoulders. Some people say that they're tired because they aren't able to articulate their need to regroup and recharge. Herbs to the rescue!

Emotional Support Tonic
MAKES 4 CUPS

These herbs help to support and condition your overworked nervous system and adrenal glands. The nettle is extracted in vinegar to obtain more of the minerals, while the others are alcohol-based tinctures. The honey adds sweetness. Depending on how you want to use this tonic (it makes a delicious salad dressing), you may choose not to add the honey.

CONTINUES →

2½ cups nettle-infused vinegar

4 tablespoons eleuthero tincture

2 tablespoons ashwagandha tincture

2 tablespoons astragalus tincture

½ cup honey (optional)

1. In a 1-quart jar, put the nettle-infused vinegar, the eleuthero, ashwagandha, and astragalus tinctures; and the honey (if using).

2. Cover and shake well to dissolve the honey.

3. Take 1½ dropperfuls in the earlier part of the day, either added to a small glass of water or straight.

4. Store the tonic at room temperature, where it will last indefinitely.

> **Tip:** I like to add a shot (about 1½ ounces) to my water bottle and drink it in the morning. It may take a couple of weeks before you notice a difference, but the ashwagandha and eleuthero can almost immediately improve your energy. True tonic herbs, nettle and astragalus work a bit slower.

Energy Decoction
MAKES 1 CUP

I love this for days when there are so many tasks looming that it is way too tempting to just crawl back under the covers and give up. It is not very tasty, but the addition of honey and lemon helps, and I usually mix it with pineapple juice or some other strongly flavored juice. It gives me energy and stamina to chew through the list of intimidating jobs!

1 teaspoon ashwagandha

1 teaspoon rhodiola

1 teaspoon eleuthero root

2 cups water

Honey (optional)

1. In a saucepan over medium-high heat, combine the ashwagandha, rhodiola, eleuthero, and water. Simmer until the mixture is reduced to half (1 cup), about 20 minutes.

2. Strain the decoction into a mug. Sweeten with honey (if using).

3. Alternatively, add half of the decoction to 16 to 32 ounces of water or juice and drink during the day.

Rise-and-Shine Bath Blend
MAKES ENOUGH FOR 1 BATH

Usually you think of baths as something soothing and relaxing, but in this case, you get an energizing bath, which is optimal for waking you up in the morning (if you have the time)! Regardless, avoid taking this stimulating bath before bedtime.

1 small muslin bag

1 tablespoon fresh or dried rosemary

1 tablespoon grated fresh ginger root

1. In a muslin bag, put the rosemary and ginger. Tie off the bag.

2. Draw a very warm but not-too-hot bath. Add the muslin tea bag to the tub.

3. Before jumping into the tub, put some of your favorite music on so you can sing along.

4. Enjoy the bath for 15 minutes or until the water cools.

5. Rinse your body and dry off briskly with a thick towel.

6. Face the day!

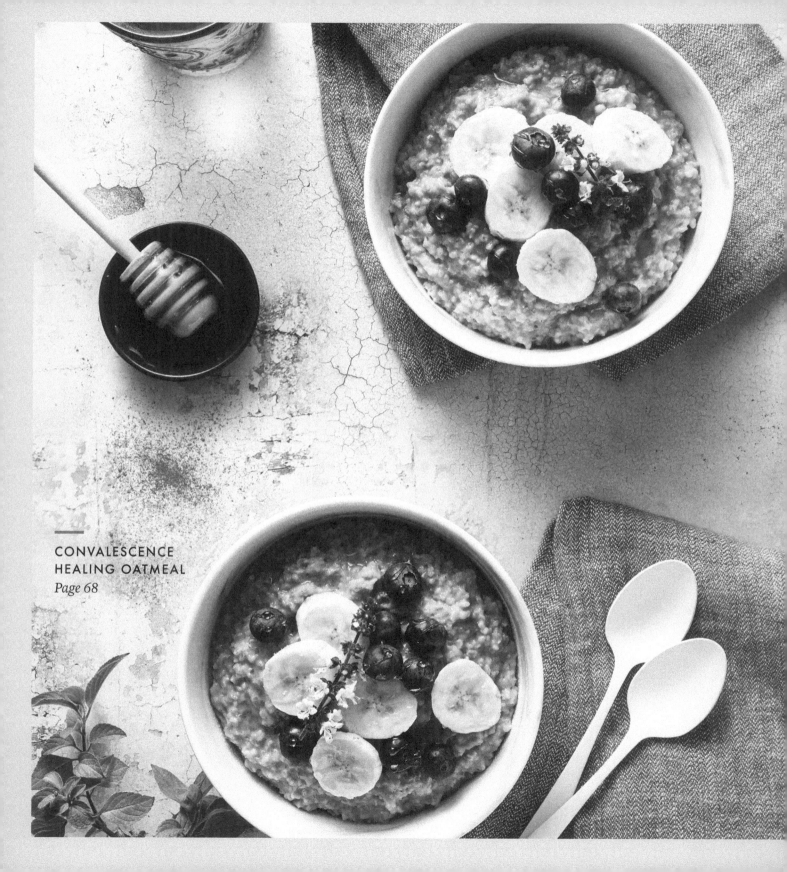

CONVALESCENCE
HEALING OATMEAL
Page 68

CHAPTER 6

Heartbreak and Grief

Nobody goes through life without experiencing the emotions of heartbreak and grief at some point. These emotions signal a period of deep sadness, and often we add in a load of guilt and a boatload of "what ifs." It can seem like the world is going on around you and you're on the outside looking in. Some people feel physical pain in their heart, and we've all heard stories of elderly couples who die within hours of each other, when the spouse left behind dies of a broken heart.

Here in Pennslyvania Dutch country, the attitude is to keep a stiff upper lip. Luckily, that seems to be changing as the older generations pass on, but grief is hard, and ignoring it just makes it last longer. It doesn't matter if it's a parent, a romantic partner, a child, or a pet, each person reacts differently to it, and all of those manifestations are valid. Herbs allies can lend support.

Caregiving

The role of caregiver, especially when a patient is at the end of life, is one of the most difficult things that many of us will ever have to do. Emotionally, we struggle with the combination of grief for the patient as well as grieving for our own lives that are pretty much taken up with this task. It can be lonely, and scary, and it can be compounded by feelings of guilt and inadequacy. Fortunately, this is an area where herbs really shine.

Convalescence Healing Oatmeal
4 SERVINGS

We think of convalescence for the patient, but here's something that can support both the patient *and* the caregiver. It's not only nutritive and nourishing, it's also filling!

For the infusion

2 cups water

2 tablespoons holy basil

3 or 4 astragalus slices

For the oatmeal

1 cup steel-cut oats

2 cups herbal infusion

1 cup milk (any kind)

Pinch salt

1 tablespoon cinnamon

Honey (optional, for topping)

Bananas (optional, for topping)

Berries (optional, for topping)

To make the infusion

1. In a small saucepan, bring the water to boil.

2. Add the holy basil and astragalus slices.

3. Cover, turn off heat, and steep for 15 minutes.

4. Strain into a bowl and add enough water to bring the mixture back up to 2 cups.

5. Set the liquid aside.

To make the oatmeal

1. In a medium saucepan, combine the oats, herbal infusion, milk, salt, and cinnamon.

2. Bring the mixture to a boil and then reduce the heat to low.

3. Simmer, uncovered, for 15 to 20 minutes until you achieve the desired thickness, stirring occasionally.

4. If the patient needs a more soupy texture, add warm milk after the oatmeal is cooked.

5. Allow to cool. If using, serve with a drizzle of honey and sliced (or mashed) bananas and berries.

6. Leftover oatmeal can be reheated but may need a little additional liquid.

Tip: If time is an issue, use plain water in place of the infusion and add a teaspoon each of astragalus and holy basil tinctures to the pot while cooking.

Holy Grail Tincture
MAKES 2 OUNCES

This blend has worked miracles for me, and I share it every chance I get. I was caring for a terminally ill sibling, which took several hours a day and near-constant supervision. At the same time, I was watching the last years of my daughter being at home slip through my fingers. I was spinning through several emotions all the time, and none of them were pleasant. Holy basil came up on a discussion board, so I mixed it with mimosa and expected nothing. About 15 minutes later, I noticed that tears were no longer rolling down my cheeks. Somehow, my struggles were moved off to the side so I could look at them from a safe distance and not drown in them.

2 tablespoons holy basil tincture

2 tablespoons mimosa tincture

1. In a measuring cup, combine the holy basil and mimosa tinctures.

2. Transfer the mixture into a 2-ounce dropper bottle.

3. Label and date the tincture blend.

4. Take 1 to 2 dropperfuls (25 to 50 drops) in 1 ounce of water or juice up to 4 times a day.

5. Store the tincture blend in a cool, dark place, where it will last for several years.

Headache

As if being depressed isn't rough enough, those tears often come with a headache. No matter if it's from trying to hold back tears or from big, breathless sobs, muscle tension and stuffed sinuses conspire to make things worse.

Headache from Crying Tea Blend
15 (1-CUP) SERVINGS

Nice hot tea hitting the palate helps relax the muscles and soothe the sinuses. The herbs in this blend relax and help clear your head.

¼ cup chamomile

¼ cup peppermint

1 fresh ginger root slice per cup (for serving)

Honey (optional)

1. In a small bowl, combine the chamomile and peppermint.

2. Transfer the tea blend to an airtight container. Label and date the blend.

3. To prepare, place a slice of fresh ginger in the bottom of a 10-ounce mug.

4. Add 1 rounded teaspoon to an infuser and place in the mug.

5. Cover with just-boiled water and steep for 3 to 5 minutes. Remove the infuser.

6. Sweeten with honey (if using).

7. Enjoy liberally.

8. Store in a cool, dry place out of direct sunlight. This will keep for a year.

Sinus Steam
MAKES ENOUGH FOR 1 STEAM

Healing warm steam laced with penetrating, soothing herbs combined with a few minutes to yourself is another way to approach healing a headache.

2 tablespoons lavender   4 cups water

2 tablespoons cup
peppermint

1. In a heatproof bowl, place the lavender and peppermint.

2. Separately, heat the water to almost boiling.

3. Place the bowl on a table where you can sit close to it.

4. Pour the water over the herbs in the bowl.

5. Sit with a towel around your shoulders and lean over the bowl.

6. Pull the towel up over your head to create a tent to contain the steam so that you are breathing it in.

Tip: I have mild claustrophobia and do not like having steams this way. I just do it without the towel and find that it is still very effective.

Oh, My Heart

Stress on the body during grief and sorrow can cause periods of heart palpitations and feeling a little out of control. As the waves of memories or emotions hit us, the body can react in surprising ways. The following recipes can support the heart and nerves that get a workout during grief. Note: Never ignore chest pain or difficulty breathing. They require immediate medical attention.

Palpitation Tea Blend
20 (1-CUP) SERVINGS

These herbs are pleasant in a tea, and the act of stopping and taking time for a cup of tea is conducive to pulling back to a more centered and grounded place. This tea is equal parts of the three herbs. If it would be easier to comply with taking a tincture, just use that proportion to create a tincture. Either preparation is equally effective.

¼ cup hawthorn
berries, leaves,
and flowers

2 tablespoons
milky oats

¼ cup ginkgo

2 tablespoons oatstraw

1. In a small bowl, combine the hawthorn, oatstraw and milky oats, and ginkgo.

2. Transfer the tea blend to an airtight container. Label and date the blend.

3. To use, add 1 rounded teaspoon to an infuser and place in a 10-ounce mug.

4. Cover with just-boiled water and steep for 5 to 7 minutes. Remove the infuser.

5. Drink 1 to 2 cups per day.

6. Store in a cool, dry place out of direct sunlight. This will keep for a year.

Heart Balm Tincture
MAKES 4 OUNCES

Help for the heart and soul are here. This soothing and calming tincture can be helpful for various types of upset in addition to palpitation. It is relaxing to the nerves while supporting and loving the heart.

3 tablespoons hawthorn tincture	1 tablespoon passionflower tincture
3 tablespoons motherwort tincture	1 tablespoon rose tincture

1. In a measuring cup, combine the hawthorn, motherwort, passionflower, and rose tinctures.

2. Transfer the mixture into a 4-ounce dropper bottle.

3. Label and date the tincture blend.

4. Take 1 dropperful (25 to 30 drops) in 1 ounce of water or juice up to 4 times a day.

5. Store the tincture blend in a cool, dark place, where it will last for several years.

Overwhelm

It always seems like when things start rolling downhill, they keep finding ways to get worse. Really, if we were in a better frame of mind, we'd know that isn't really true, but when we're overwhelmed, it's hard to see things clearly. Here are a few options to stop that snowball before it gets any bigger. Maybe we can even melt it!

Nervous Exhaustion Tonic
MAKES 4 OUNCES

If facing a long-term situation seems like "too much," a daily tonic with some adaptogens is a good proactive approach.

2 tablespoons milky oats tincture	2 tablespoons eleuthero tincture
2 tablespoons passionflower tincture	2 tablespoons astragalus tincture

1. In a measuring cup, combine the milky oats, passionflower, eleuthero, and astragalus tinctures.

2. Transfer the mixture into a 4-ounce dropper bottle.

3. Label and date the tincture blend.

4. Take 1 to 2 dropperfuls (25 to 50 drops) in 1 ounce of water or juice 1 or 2 times per day.

5. Store the tincture blend in a cool, dark place, where it will last for several years.

Bathtub, Take Me Away Blend
MAKES ENOUGH FOR 16 BATHS

Slip into a warm bath scented and embellished with these comforting additions. Epsom salt is so good for relaxing tense muscles, and these herbs along with the milk soothe your skin while smoothing out your emotions.

1 cup rose

1 cup elderflowers

1 cup milk powder (any kind of milk)

1 cup Epsom salt

1. In a large bowl, combine the rose, elder-flowers, milk powder, and Epsom salt.

2. Transfer the tea blend to an airtight container. Label and date the blend.

3. To use, place about ¼ cup of the blend in a muslin bag or an infuser.

4. Place the muslin bag with the herb mixture in a heat-resistant container and cover with just-boiled water.

5. Steep the bath tea while drawing the bath.

6. Pour the bath tea into the tub and climb in.

7. Soak and relax for at least 15 minutes.

8. Store in a cool, dry place out of direct sunlight. This will keep for a year.

Tip: If there's no powdered milk in the house, substitute 2 cups of liquid milk poured right into the tub with each bath. If you don't have a muslin bag or infuser, a sock can be used in a pinch, tied to enclose the mixture.

Resilience Tincture
MAKES 4 OUNCES

With this tincture, you're getting something that can help you handle everything the world is doling out right now. A tall order? Yes it is. Rest, immune system support, and pain relief all conspire to increase your resilience, giving you the ability to take it all on—tomorrow.

3 tablespoons California poppy tincture

3 tablespoons blue vervain tincture

1 tablespoon holy basil tincture

1 tablespoon elderberry tincture

1. In a measuring cup, combine the California poppy, blue vervain, holy basil, and elderberry tinctures.

2. Transfer the mixture into a 4-ounce dropper bottle.

3. Label and date the tincture blend.

4. Take 25 to 40 drops in 1 ounce of water or juice in the evening, preferably after a warm bath.

5. Store the tincture blend in a cool, dark place, where it will last for several years.

Sleep Disruptions or Altered Dreams

Heartbreak and grief can bring up a lot of unconscious worries. How will this change the future? Will life ever be normal again? All kinds of questions and concerns are floating around in our brain, just waiting to turn up in a dream or wake us up to fret. Magnesium supplements or Epsom salt baths help smooth everything out. Reading a book (a physical book, not an e-book on a screen) just before bed that isn't too stimulating or scary can help put your brain in a good place for sleep.

Sweet Dreams Pillow
MAKES 1 PILLOW

You don't always have to ingest herbs or put them on your body for them to be healing. In this case, aromatherapy through the soothing scent of lavender sets a calming bedtime scene. This small sachet can be slipped under your pillow or kept on a bedside table.

9-by-13-inch piece of heavy flannel cloth   **2 cups lavender**

1. Fold the cloth in half with the right side in so that the size is 9 inches by 6½ inches.

2. Sew one of the short ends and the other long end, leaving about ½-inch seam allowance.

3. Turn the sack inside out.

4. Fill with the lavender.

5. Sew shut the remaining short end.

6. Keep the pillow sachet near the head of your bed where the fragrance can be inhaled.

> **Tip:** Lavender continues to exude fragrance until it is ground to dust—and even the dust is fragrant!

Sleep Potion
MAKES 4 OUNCES

Formulated to quiet those recurring worries and thoughts, gently sedate, and make sleep less elusive, this potion will become a great ally to those who suffer from insomnia. If you're prone to waking up in the middle of the night and not being able to get back to sleep, I recommend keeping a dose of this mixed in a couple of ounces of water in a glass by your bed.

4 tablespoons California poppy tincture   **2 tablespoons lavender-infused honey**

2 tablespoons passionflower tincture

CONTINUES →

1. In a measuring cup, combine the California poppy and passionflower tinctures. Add the honey and mix well to combine.

2. Transfer the mixture into a 4-ounce dropper bottle.

3. Label and date the tincture blend.

4. Take 30 to 40 drops shortly before bed.

5. Store the tincture blend in a cool, dark place, where it will last for several years.

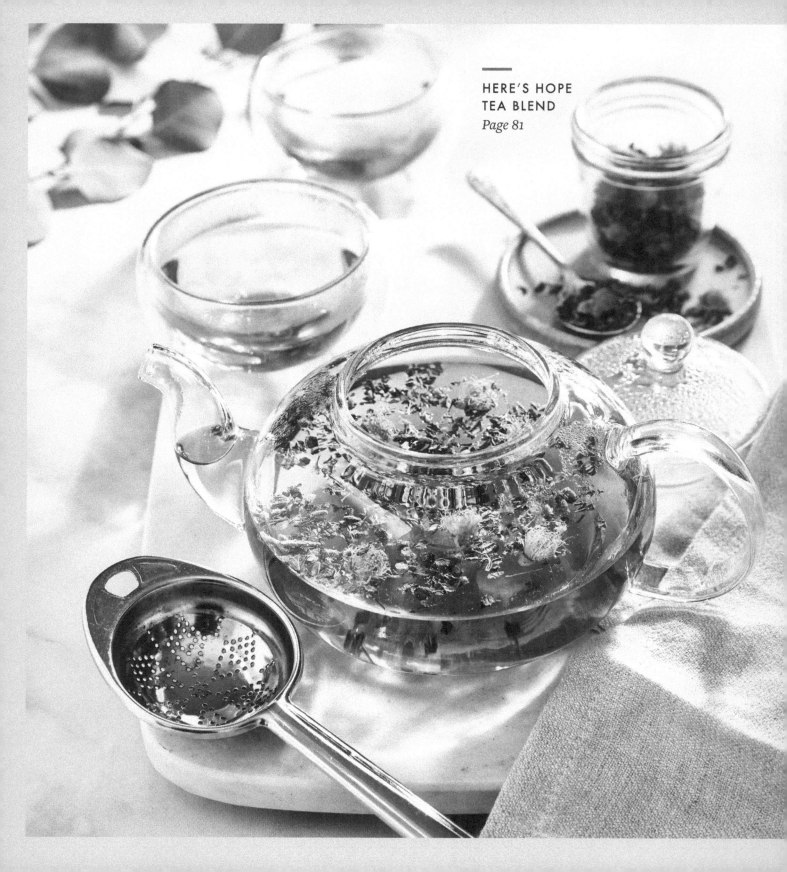

HERE'S HOPE
TEA BLEND
Page 81

CHAPTER 7

Powerlessness, Resentment, Regret, and Guilt

Fear, anger, and feelings of inadequacy spring from these conditions. You might recognize this most easily in elderly patients who fight their caregivers and are fearful or suspicious. Unfortunately, this energy seems to be very contagious, and being around someone who is feeling this way can drag you down as well. And sometimes you may be the one experiencing these constricting emotions. Herbs, exercise, sunshine, meditation, and mindfulness can all bring about self-awareness so you can start to see things in a different, more positive perspective.

Aches and Pains

In addition to being more susceptible to feeling pain from autoimmune flare-ups and irregular rest (among many other causes), all of a sudden you may be hyper-focused on every little thing. It may seem counterproductive, but as long as a medical condition isn't in the way, this is precisely when exercise, yoga, tai chi, or simple walks can help ease pain. If you can enlist a friend to help keep you on track, it may even become a favorite part of your day.

Aches and Pains Tincture

MAKES 4 OUNCES

This is a great combination. In addition to helping relieve pain, it can ease you to into sleep, and it also has antidepressant properties.

3 tablespoons skullcap tincture

2 tablespoons valerian tincture

3 tablespoons blue vervain tincture

1. In a measuring cup, combine the skullcap, blue vervain, and valerian tinctures.

2. Transfer the mixture into a 4-ounce dropper bottle.

3. Label and date the tincture blend.

4. Take 1 dropperful (25 drops) in 1 ounce of water or juice as needed.

5. Store the tincture blend in a cool, dark place, where it will last for several years.

Sore Muscles and Cramp Oil

MAKES 5 OUNCES

If you're experiencing a problem with muscle cramping, be sure you're getting enough magnesium and calcium. Magnesium citrate is a very effective form, but it works as a laxative, so if that's an issue, the more readily available oxide and glycinate forms are preferable. Taking an Epsom salt bath is another good way to get magnesium, as is eating magnesium-rich foods, such as dark chocolate. Massaging this herbal oil into your sore muscles also provides relief.

½ cup lavender-infused olive oil

2 tablespoons rosemary-infused olive oil

1. Pour the lavender- and rosemary-infused olive oils into an unbreakable bottle with a flip top that controls the flow.

2. Massage into skin as needed.

3. Store in a cool, dark place, and use within 6 months.

Tip: In this case, it's best to use a plastic bottle; glass bottles used to store oils can become slippery, and you risk the bottle falling and breaking.

Gotcha in the Gut

We sometimes say that something is "eating away at us." You'll feel that in your gut as well as in your heart and emotions, and it can really hurt! The smooth muscle that makes up most of your digestive system can cramp or spasm. You can relax those muscles (and protect the mucus membrane lining from the effects of excess stomach acid) with soothing, slick, mucilaginous plants. Try these remedies for relief.

Cramp Drops

MAKES 2 OUNCES

One of the most prevalent symptoms of emotional upset is intestinal cramping. This tincture blend helps relax your muscles. Note that this blend can also be made into a tea by substituting dried herbs, but valerian root tea tastes very bitter. So, drop the valerian, use equal parts of the other three herbs, and add a slice of fresh ginger to each cup of tea.

1 tablespoon catnip tincture	1 tablespoon peppermint tincture
1 tablespoon chamomile tincture	1 tablespoon valerian tincture

1. In a measuring cup, combine the catnip, chamomile, peppermint, and valerian tinctures.

2. Transfer the mixture into a 2-ounce dropper bottle.

3. Label and date the tincture blend.

4. Take 15 to 20 drops in 1 ounce (or less) of water as needed.

5. Store the tincture blend in a cool, dark place, where it will last for several years.

Gutsy Brew

MAKES 1 QUART

If you're prone to irritable bowel syndrome (IBS) or any type of autoimmune issue that shows up in the gut, you may experience flare-ups during emotionally trying times. Of course, they can happen to anyone, so if discomfort becomes a problem, turn to this tea, which coats and soothes the gut and bowel while also toning; plantain is good for healing tissue. For this, you use a cold infusion method, so it's best made up the night before you plan to drink it.

1 tablespoon plantain	2 astragalus slices
1 tablespoon marshmallow root	1 tablespoon peppermint
1 tablespoon rose	

1. In a 1-quart jar, combine the plantain, marshmallow root, rose, astragalus, and peppermint.

2. Fill the jar with cold water.

3. Cover and place the mixture in the fridge overnight.

4. In the morning, strain, and drink throughout the day.

Internal Tapes on a Loop

We all have tapes playing in our heads. They begin in childhood, as our parents speak to us, and over time, we allow them to become our own personal soundtrack, or "self-talk." When you're feeling positive about life, either those tapes are telling you good things or you're able to quiet negative stories. However, when you are struggling with bitterness and resentment, these tapes can become self-defeating, encouraging you to cling to memories of injustice and think less of yourself. The best thing you can do during those times is to turn down the volume on those tapes as much as possible. When you're feeling stronger, you can take a closer look at what you tell yourself and work on revising those stories.

Let It Go Toddy
2 SERVINGS

Particularly nice on a cold winter night, this twist on a classic comforting drink is very flexible and can be easily altered by making an infusion with the hot water, using infused honey, or completely swapping out the herbs. This recipe is meant to be shared. If only one person will be drinking it, halve the recipe.

1½ cups hot water

1 tablespoon honey

2 tablespoons lavender-infused vinegar

1 tablespoon hawthorn tincture

1 tablespoon lemon balm tincture

2 lemon wedges

1. In a measuring cup, combine the water, honey, and lavender-infused vinegar. Mix well to combine.

2. Add the hawthorn and lemon balm tinctures and combine.

3. Divide the mixture into two teacups.

4. Garnish with a wedge of lemon and enjoy warm.

Turn Off the Reruns Formula
MAKES 4 OUNCES

Remember that time when you were nine years old and the neighbor caught you picking her tulips? Or how about that time in gym class when you couldn't keep up, so you lied about an injury? Remember that time when you broke someone's heart? All the cringe-worthy moments in life seem to be sitting on a shelf in your brain, just waiting to torment you—usually for no apparent reason. This combination of herbs works to stop incessant internal chatter and give your brain a rest.

2 tablespoons passionflower tincture

2 tablespoons St. John's wort tincture

1 tablespoon ashwagandha tincture

1 tablespoon valerian tincture

2 tablespoons milky oats–infused vinegar

1. In a measuring cup, combine the passion-flower, St. John's wort, ashwagandha, and valerian tinctures. Add the milky oats–infused vinegar and combine well.

2. Pour the mixture into a 4-ounce dropper bottle (or two 2-ounce dropper bottles).

3. Label and date the bottles.

4. Take 25 to 30 drops up to 3 times a day.

5. Store in a cool, dark place, where it will last for several years.

Smile Mimosa Drops
30 SERVINGS

Did you know that smiling facial muscles release endorphins, which can make you happy? I learned this in one of my first alternative healing classes in the mid-'90s, and since then I've read many studies showing that smiling also improves immunity and lowers stress and depression! It's a "fake it 'til you make it" thing: Your brain doesn't differentiate between a "real" smile and the action. Known as "the tree of happiness," mimosa provides support to get you to the real thing.

2 tablespoons mimosa tincture

1. Add 25 drops of mimosa tincture to your morning tea.

2. Add another 25 drops to a water bottle and drink during the day.

3. Remember to smile, not for anyone but yourself.

> **Tip:** A full 1-ounce bottle dropper holds 25 to 30 drops. Each 1-ounce bottle contains 30 dropperfuls of tincture.

Here's Hope Tea Blend
15 (1-CUP) SERVINGS

I love this blend. It really lightens a heavy mood. It also tastes delicious with a little dab of honey!

¼ cup lemon balm   **1 tablespoon lavender**

¼ cup mimosa bark (or flowers if available)

1. In a large bowl, combine the lemon balm, mimosa, and lavender.

2. Transfer the tea blend to an airtight container. Label and date the blend.

3. To use, add 1 rounded teaspoon to an infuser and place in a 10-ounce mug.

4. Cover with just-boiled water and steep for 5 to 7 minutes. Remove the infuser.

5. Drink 1 or 2 cups per day.

6. Store in a cool, dry place out of direct sunlight. This will keep for a year.

Irritabili-Tea Blend

40 (1-CUP) SERVINGS

One of the things I like about this blend is that it also gives your immune system a hand, something that can be needed when you're under emotional strain. My family drinks a lot of it around here in the winter as a preventive for both immunity and grouchiness.

½ **cup holy basil**

¼ **cup mimosa bark**

¼ **cup lemon balm**

2 **tablespoons elderberries**

2 **tablespoons rose**

1. In a medium bowl, combine the holy basil, mimosa bark, lemon balm, elderberries, and rose.

2. Transfer the tea blend to an airtight container. Label and date the blend.

3. To use, add 1 rounded teaspoon to an infuser and place in a 10-ounce mug.

4. Cover with just-boiled water and steep for 5 to 7 minutes. Remove the infuser.

5. Drink 1 or 2 cups a day.

6. Store in a cool, dry place out of direct sunlight. This will keep for a year.

New Perspective Tincture

MAKES 2 OUNCES

Being cranky is a self-fulfilling mood because it makes other people either avoid us or snap back. Changing the way you look at things can be such a gift when you're in a bad head-space. This tincture blend gently leads you to a brighter outlook.

2 **tablespoons skullcap tincture**

2 **tablespoons motherwort tincture**

1. In a measuring cup, combine the skull-cap and motherwort tinctures.

2. Transfer the mixture into a 2-ounce dropper bottle.

3. Label and date the tincture blend.

4. Take 1 dropperful (25 to 30 drops) as needed up to 3 times a day.

5. Store the tincture blend in a cool, dark place, where it will last for several years.

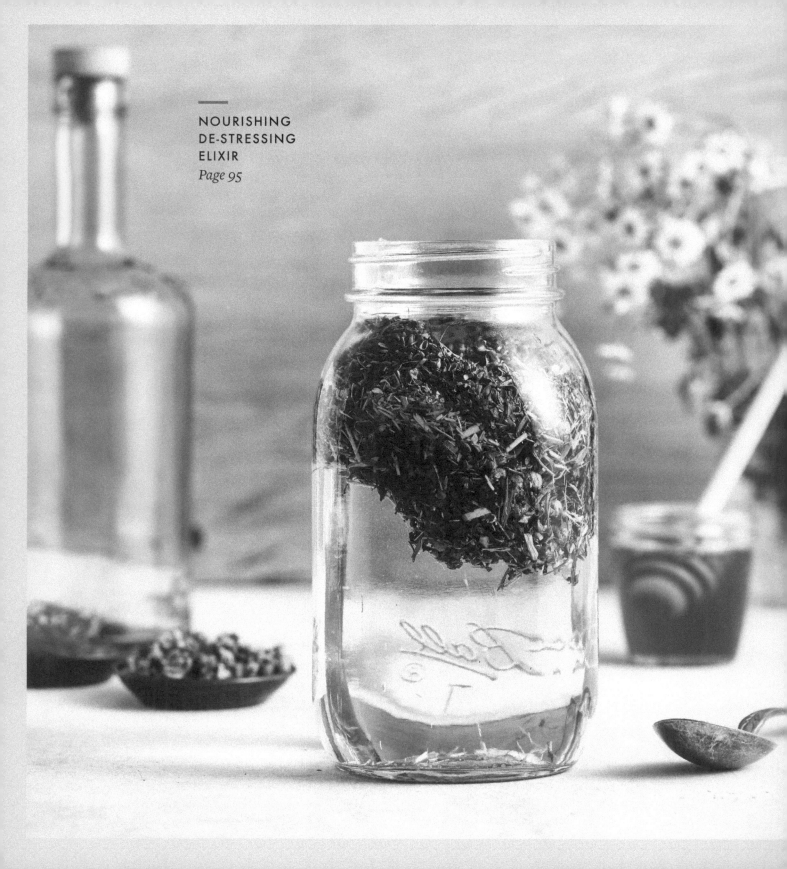

NOURISHING
DE-STRESSING
ELIXIR
Page 95

CHAPTER 8

Stress

Stress leads to many other emotional conditions and states. Everyone has some degree of stress in their lives. It is part of the human condition. Stress, and how you handle it physically, emotionally, and spiritually, often determines your mental health. You can look for the root of the stress and try to get to the bottom of that issue while employing such tools as breathing, meditation, yoga, acupressure, and exercise so you're in a position of strength when facing it. In addition, there are powerful allies in the plant world, and they can help quite a bit.

When stressed, we enter into a "fight-or-flight" response, a leftover from our prehistoric days of survival of the fittest. As modern humans, we struggle to contain these reactions, which is even more stressful! If you want to remain employed, you can't run or start a fight when your boss calls you into her office. When something stressful occurs, like a car accident, most people successfully manage to stay somewhat calm—and resist the urge to run away. However, that doesn't mean that your body isn't still reacting with that primal "fight-or-flight" response; after all, your system *is* flooded with adrenaline and cortisol! Your heart beats faster, raising your blood pressure, which in turn flows to your lungs, muscles, and trunk, while restricting flow to the extremities. You breathe harder and faster, pulling in oxygen to take on any perceived threat. You're ready for anything.

Sometimes, stress is positive. It enables us to react quickly to real threats. We've all heard stories about people performing superhuman feats to save someone during an emergency. New parents need that stress to be alert for the new little person for whom they're responsible. Stress might get us through job interviews and college finals. Personally, I love the stress of deadlines and need it to keep my life under control. For me, that's stress in all its glory.

When the threat passes, you calm down fairly quickly and go about your life. But sometimes the threats happen too often. Sometimes stress is constant. When you can't bounce back, the stress response can cause physical damage and erode your emotional wellness. Stress affects all of your organs, all of your senses, and even your thoughts and dreams. If only for your quality of life, stress shouldn't be given the upper hand. We'll call on the herbs for support.

Balance and Stability

It may be surprising to learn that those periods of clumsiness, bumping into things, and feeling unsteady can be related to stress. It can be that stress is messing with your nerves, which play an important role in helping you maintain balance and solid footing. One of the clearest examples of this that a lot of people experience is a nerve conduction study, often used to determine if carpal tunnel syndrome is present. Electrodes are attached, the median nerve is stimulated, and the reaction is observed. It's easy to imagine how easily the impulses throughout the body can be slowed or short-circuited by the many different hormones, toxic waste products, and chemicals that our bodies produce during stressful times.

Be sure to get plenty of fluids and nourishment. Deep breathing is also important. The following blends are intended to help blood flow and awareness and keep any nausea (similar to motion sickness) at bay.

Balanced and Secure Tincture
MAKES 2 OUNCES

In college, I really screwed up on a deadline, and my professor was not offering any flexibility. It was a final paper, and the whole thing was very upsetting. It coincided with a romantic breakup. Ugh. I started to notice that when I stood in the hall waiting for class, the floor and walls were "wavy." Of course they weren't. I was just very stressed about that class. At that age, I didn't have any relaxation tools, nor did I have any knowledge of herbs that could help. When I look back, I think this tincture would have been a big help.

1 tablespoon ashwagandha tincture

1 tablespoon catnip tincture

1 tablespoon ginkgo tincture

½ tablespoon ginger root tincture

½ tablespoon holy basil tincture

1. In a measuring cup, combine the ashwagandha, catnip, ginkgo, ginger, and holy basil tinctures.

2. Transfer the mixture into a 2-ounce dropper bottle.

3. Label and date the tincture blend.

4. Take 1 dropperful (25 to 30 drops) in 1 ounce of water as needed up to 3 times a day.

5. Store the tincture blend in a cool, dark place, where it will last for several years.

Dizzy in a Tizzy Tea Blend
35 (1-CUP) SERVINGS

Running around in circles? Bumping into things? Maybe a little clumsy and out of balance? Put on the kettle and have a seat!

¼ cup ginkgo

¼ cup catnip

¼ cup chamomile

2 tablespoons rosemary

2 tablespoons rose

2 tablespoons ginger root

1 tablespoon rhodiola

Honey (optional)

Lemon (optional)

1. In a bowl, combine the ginkgo, catnip, chamomile, rosemary, rose, ginger, and rhodiola.

2. Transfer the tea blend to an airtight container. Label and date the blend.

3. To use, add 1 rounded teaspoon to an infuser and place in a 10-ounce mug.

4. Cover with just-boiled water and steep for at least 5 minutes. Remove the infuser.

5. Sweeten with honey and lemon (if using).

6. Stop thinking for a few minutes while you enjoy your tea.

7. Store in a cool, dry place out of direct sunlight. This will keep for a year.

Body Tension

In stressful situations, it is easy to unconsciously hold the tension in your body. Yoga, massage, and meditation can all increase your awareness of this habit. At one time, a relative of mine would spend a day getting unpleasant—but needed—medical tests. As the day wore on, his shoulders would get closer and closer to his ears. I'd say, "Drop your shoulders," and I'm certain that he thought I was just being a nag, but I was merely trying to help him see how his body was responding to stress.

Most of the herbal preparations to ease body tension taste bitter, so tinctures are the easiest way to take them.

Balm for Sore Lips

MAKES 3 (½-OUNCE) TINS OR TUBES

A very common habit during times of stress involves licking, chewing, or pulling on the lips. It's right up there with biting the nails. It's very simple to make a soothing and mild lip balm. This recipe makes three ½-ounce tubes so you can stash them in all your bags and never be without.

¾ teaspoon beeswax pastilles

1 tablespoon lavender-infused olive oil

1 tablespoon peppermint-infused olive oil

1 tablespoon plantain-infused olive oil

1. In a heatproof bowl set over a pot ⅓ full of water, add the beeswax and the lavender-, peppermint-, and plantain-infused olive oils.

2. Over low heat, stir gently until the beeswax has liquefied and blended with the oil.

3. Pour out carefully into 3 lip balm tins or tubes.

4. Apply to chapped or sore lips as needed.

Foot Soak, Two Ways

MAKES ENOUGH FOR 1 SOAK

Most of the time, when your feet hurt, you hurt all over. It's easy to see when people are struggling with a lack of energy or when their spirits are sinking. Their bodies sink into their hips, and they slog along on feet that aren't happy. Luckily, a 15- or 20-minute foot soak can turn things around. You'll need a sturdy vessel large enough for your feet and a gallon or two of water. Stop in at a craft store and purchase a bag of marbles that would typically be used in vases to hold stems (among other uses). They'll add a massage to the soak!

For a daytime pick-me-up

1½ tablespoon rosemary

1½ tablespoon mint

1 small slice of fresh ginger root or ¼ teaspoon dried

Marbles (optional)

For a relaxing evening soak

1 tablespoon lavender	1 tablespoon
1 tablespoon plantain	St. John's wort

1. Prepare the herbs by putting them in a muslin bag.

2. Make a strong tea by pouring at least 1 quart of boiled water over the packet of herbs in a heatproof container.

3. If using, place the marbles on the bottom of the foot soak container.

4. Fill the container about ½ full with room-temperature water.

5. Add the hot tea.

6. Adjust the temperature by adding cool water if necessary.

7. While soaking, rub the soles of your feet on the marbles. It's amazing how they can work kinks out of feet that have been warmed in water for a few minutes.

8. When finished, rinse the marbles well so they're ready for the next time.

Head and Shoulders Tension Tincture

MAKES 2 OUNCES

When you are stressed, you clench your jaw, hunch your shoulders toward your ears, and keep your tongue tight to the top of your mouth. After a while, this can result in a sore jaw, possibly chipped teeth, and a painful neck and shoulders. The Herbal Hot Pad (page 44) used alongside this tincture can ease tension and promote relaxation.

2 tablespoons skullcap tincture	½ tablespoon valerian tincture
1 tablespoon passionflower tincture	½ tablespoon blue vervain tincture

1. In a measuring cup, combine the skullcap, passionflower, valerian, and blue vervain tinctures.

2. Transfer the mixture into a 2-ounce dropper bottle.

3. Label and date the tincture blend.

4. Take 1 dropperful (25 to 30 drops) in 1 ounce of water or juice as needed. Repeat the dose 30 minutes later if needed.

5. Store the tincture blend in a cool, dark place, where it will last for several years.

My Aching Back Tincture

MAKES 2 OUNCES

A lot of times, stress hits me as a muscle spasm in the lower back. It can completely gum up the works, and that just adds to the stress. This is another good use for the Herbal Hot Pad (page 44) at the first hint

CONTINUES →

of muscle spasms. Add this tincture and try some stretches that are specifically meant to strengthen the core and relax the spasms. The herbs in this blend combine to relax and relieve pain and muscle spasms.

1 tablespoon blue vervain tincture

1 tablespoon motherwort tincture

1 tablespoon valerian tincture

1 tablespoon skullcap tincture

1. In a measuring cup, combine the blue vervain, valerian, motherwort, and skullcap tinctures.

2. Transfer the mixture into a 2-ounce dropper bottle.

3. Label and date the tincture blend.

4. Take 1 dropperful (25 to 30 drops) in 1 ounce of water or juice as needed. Repeat the dose 30 minutes later if needed up to 4 times to obtain relief.

5. Store the tincture blend in a cool, dark place, where it will last for several years.

Tics and Muscular Cramps Drops
MAKES 2 OUNCES

Most people have experienced twitches at the corners of the eyes when overworked or stressed out. Other muscles aren't always as obvious, but they can also develop tics and cramps. These symptoms are a good indication that it's time to take a break, find a different solution to the problem at hand, or prioritize

rest. Of course, rest is the last thing you think about when you're working so hard and under pressure. Try this tincture the next time you're overtired. It might be just the thing.

2 tablespoons California poppy tincture

2 tablespoons skullcap tincture

1. In a measuring cup, combine the California poppy and skullcap tinctures.

2. Transfer the mixture into a 2-ounce dropper bottle.

3. Label and date the tincture blend.

4. Take 1 dropperful (25 to 30 drops) as needed.

5. Store the tincture blend in a cool, dark place, where it will last for several years.

> Tip: Consider taking a relaxing bath, turning off the computer, and listening to some soothing music after taking these drops.

Build Immunity

Stress takes a toll on immunity. It stresses your body, your organs, and your built-in defense mechanisms, leaving you more vulnerable to viruses and bacterial infections. And when you're in a weakened condition, you're more susceptible to catching whatever sicknesses your coworkers bring to work with them. Handwashing and avoiding touching your face can help prevent an illness from taking hold.

I know that when I couldn't bring a virus into the house for three years, I used some of the remedies that follow and stayed healthy.

Just because colds and viruses are swirling around, it doesn't mean that you have to get them. You can create a few immune-building remedies and use one of them every day. Switch them up. Stress is just a part of life, and we never know when life is going to crank up the noise, so be prepared. Make one or more of these blends a part of your daily ritual during the winter months, and you'll find that you'll avoid bugs entirely—or, if they do take hold, you'll get better much quicker.

Antiviral Tincture
MAKES 2 OUNCES

This blend of herbs is specifically antiviral. It is one that I like to take if I feel stressed and there are viruses going around. I figure that if you have the option, why not avoid them altogether? Make this tincture part of your prevention protocol when exposure to illness is inevitable.

1 tablespoon echinacea tincture

1 tablespoon elderberry tincture

1 tablespoon lemon balm tincture

1 tablespoon thyme tincture

1. In a measuring cup, combine the echinacea, elderberry, lemon balm, and thyme tinctures.

2. Transfer the mixture into a 2-ounce dropper bottle.

3. Label and date the tincture blend.

4. Take 1 dropperful (25 to 30 drops) in 1 ounce of water or juice 4 times a day. If you will be exposed to crowds, take it preemptively.

5. Store the tincture blend in a cool, dark place, where it will last for several years.

Outbreak Tea and Spray
MAKES 8 OUNCES

Stress weakens the immune system, and being run down with a weakened immune system makes us easy targets for a variety of painful outbreaks. One such virus, shingles (herpes zoster), seems to be more and more common. I once came down with shingles after a pretty intense period of work. I tried dozens of things, but one of the most effective for temporary relief of the pain was a combination of these herbs made into a spray. I particularly liked it because I didn't need to touch the rash to apply it!

1¼ cups water

2 tablespoons St. John's wort

2 tablespoons lemon balm

1. In a small pot, heat the water to boiling. Once boiling, turn off the heat.

2. Add the St. John's wort and lemon balm and steep for about 30 minutes.

CONTINUES →

3. Strain the mixture through a very fine-mesh strainer and/or cloth (like an old T-shirt).

4. Pour the liquid into a spray bottle and keep it in the refrigerator.

5. Throw the spray away when the outbreak is gone.

> **Tip:** If the chilled spray is annoying to your skin, keep most of it in the fridge and fill a 1-ounce spray bottle that stays out for use. Alternatively, add 1 ounce of alcohol to preserve the 8 ounces.

Sore Throat Syrup
MAKES 12 OUNCES

Often the very first signs of impending illness or lowered immunity are swollen glands and a sore throat. This syrup is very effective at calming things down. It's a go-to remedy at our house. In a real pinch, simple sage tea with lemon and honey also works amazingly well.

1 tablespoon marshmallow root	1 tablespoon echinacea root
½ cup cool water	½ cup honey
1 tablespoon sage	Salt water (optional)

1. Begin the cold infusion: cover the marshmallow root with the cool water and steep it at room temperature (or in the fridge) for a few hours.

2. Steep the sage and echinacea in 5 ounces of just-boiled water for 30 minutes.

3. Strain the sage and echinacea. We need 4½ ounces of this tea.

4. Add the honey and warm gently if needed to incorporate.

5. Add the marshmallow root infusion, which is about 3½ ounces.

6. Transfer the syrup into bottles. Label and date them.

7. Take by the spoonful to soothe the throat.

8. Gargle with salt water (if using) a few times a day as well.

9. Store in the refrigerator and take within a week.

> **Tip:** The exact same herbs can be blended dry and brewed as a tea. Use 1 teaspoon to a cup of just-boiled water. Add honey and lemon to taste.

Triple-Threat Tincture
MAKES 4 OUNCES

There are a handful of remedies that I am rarely without, and this is one of them. It provides such strong immune system support, and on top of that, the holy basil and astragalus are adaptogens that help your body handle stress so it doesn't contribute to weakening your immunity.

3 tablespoons elderberry tincture	2 tablespoons astragalus tincture
3 tablespoons holy basil tincture	

1. In a measuring cup, combine the elderberry, holy basil, and astragalus tinctures.

2. Transfer the mixture into a 4-ounce dropper bottle.

3. Label and date the tincture blend.

4. Take 1 to 2 dropperfuls (25 to 50 drops) each morning with breakfast or at any other time of day that is easy to remember to do regularly.

5. Store the tincture blend in a cool, dark place, where it will last for several years.

Virus, Cold, and Flu Tea Blend
35 (1-CUP) SERVINGS

For this tea, I chop the echinacea root and astragalus root small so that they will more easily infuse. They can be purchased in cut/sifted form, which is about right. This blend can become a daily beverage to help support immunity.

¼ cup echinacea root	¼ cup peppermint
¼ cup astragalus	1 heaping tablespoon thyme
¼ cup elderberries	
	Honey (optional)

1. In a large bowl, combine the echinacea, astragalus, elderberries, peppermint, and thyme.

2. Transfer the tea blend to an airtight container. Label and date the blend.

3. To use, add 1 rounded teaspoon to an infuser and place in a 10-ounce mug.

4. Cover with just-boiled water and steep for at least 5 minutes. Remove the infuser.

5. Sweeten with honey (if using).

6. Store in a cool, dry place out of direct sunlight. This will keep for a year.

General De-Stressing Remedies

Stress is a fact of life. You likely have coping mechanisms you've always used, but it's also helpful to discover ways to be proactive in cutting stress off before it gets too intense. For me, getting outside and weeding, gathering, digging, or pinching off the faded blossoms puts my head back on straight. That's my thing. Still, there are times when stress can sneak up and knock the wind out of your sails. It's so much better to have a reserve of strength built up. The following recipes are very good for that.

Additionally, find things that make you feel good. Do art. You don't have to be good because it's about expressing what's going on inside. Take a class in something you've wanted to learn. Cooking, pottery, literature, psychology—whatever you want. Herbalism is a good one. Call a friend and go for a walk. Most important, do something you want to do that makes you feel better.

Long-Term Stress Tonic Elixir
MAKES ABOUT 24 OUNCES

It's good to make a large batch of the elixir because it's so good to have on hand. We can't always quickly fix the things that cause us stress. Long-term stress can be so destructive to us physically and destroy our mood and outlook. These versatile and gentle adaptogens work together to support the body through stress that lasts for more than a few days (or weeks).

⅓ cup holy basil

¼ cup ashwagandha

¼ cup astragalus

½ cup honey

2½ cups alcohol of choice

1. To a 1-quart jar, put the holy basil, ashwagandha, and astragalus.

2. Add the honey and stir well to combine.

3. Add the alcohol and combine well. Cover the jar and shake well.

4. Infuse the elixir for at least 2 weeks, storing it in a cool, dark place and shaking occasionally.

5. Once it's done infusing, strain the elixir and transfer it to bottles.

6. Label and date the elixir.

7. Take a teaspoon each day to help keep stress-related health issues under control.

8. Store the elixir in a cool, dark place, where it will last for several years.

Nettle and Oatstraw Concentrate
MAKES 1 QUART, ENOUGH FOR 1 DAY

More than 20 years ago, I attended a conference where I listened to Susun Weed talk about making a very strong nettle infusion. The talk focused on how modern life is so hard on our adrenals, which are constantly assaulted. Since that time, these concentrated tea blends have become quite popular! They involve a small number of herbs that are nourishing and nutritive to your system. These herbs don't have strong scents (meaning the plants do not produce much, if any, essential oil); nettle, oatstraw, raspberry leaf, red clover, chickweed, and plantain are typically used.

½ cup nettle

1 cup oatstraw

1 quart water

1. Place the nettle and oatstraw in a quart canning jar.

2. Boil the water, and then pour it over the herbs in the jar.

3. Cover the jar lightly. I put a plate on top of the jar.

4. Steep until the morning.

5. Strain, pressing as much of the liquid from the herbs as possible.

6. Drink the tea throughout the day.

7. If the taste is objectionable, add it to juice.

Tip: While this can be done anytime, most people make it before bed so it's ready to drink the following morning.

Nourishing De-Stressing Elixir
MAKES 16 OUNCES

Because stress is such a universal affliction, this is a good herbal remedy to make and have on hand. This blend is dual-action—it provides instant relief and also helps build and support a healthy nervous system in the long term.

2 tablespoons holy basil

2 tablespoons lemon balm

2 tablespoons chamomile

2 tablespoons skullcap

1 tablespoon passionflower

1 tablespoon California poppy

1 tablespoon eleuthero root

¾ cup honey

3 tablespoons milky oats–infused vinegar

1 cup plus 2 tablespoons alcohol of choice

1. In a quart jar, put the holy basil, lemon balm, chamomile, skullcap, passionflower, California poppy, and eleuthero.

2. Add the honey and stir a bit to coat the herbs.

3. Add the milky oats–infused vinegar.

4. Top off with the alcohol.

5. Cover the jar and shake well.

6. Infuse the elixir for 2 to 4 weeks, storing it in a cool, dark place and shaking occasionally.

7. Once it's done infusing, strain the elixir and transfer it to dropper bottles.

8. Label and date the elixir.

9. Take it by the teaspoon 1 or 2 times a day.

10. Store the elixir in a cool, dark place, where it will be good for several years.

SOS Tea Blend

35 (1-CUP) SERVINGS

Here's a great tea to bolster the nerves from the kind of stress that is repetitious and out of nowhere. Think of first responders or new parents, for example. Those repeated surprises exhaust us, and eventually our adrenal glands are also out of whack. Support yourself, your nerves, and your adrenals with this tasty tea. This can be enjoyed as often as you like—even daily. The nettle and oats have the ability to build, repair, and nourish the nerves, while the other herbs are more immediate. Add 15 minutes outside in fresh air and nature, and you might feel like a brand-new person.

¼ **cup eleuthero root**

¼ **cup nettle**

¼ **cup holy basil**

2 tablespoons milky oats

2 tablespoons ashwagandha

2 tablespoons lemon balm

Honey (optional)

1. In a bowl, combine the eleuthero, nettle, holy basil, milky oats, ashwagandha, and lemon balm.

2. Transfer the tea blend to an airtight container. Label and date the blend.

3. To use, add 1 rounded teaspoon to an infuser and place in a 10-ounce mug.

4. Cover with just-boiled water and steep for 5 to 7 minutes. Remove the infuser.

5. Sweeten with honey (if using).

6. Enjoy liberally.

7. Store in a cool, dry place out of direct sunlight. This will keep for a year.

Headaches

There are so many ways that stress can give us headaches. We clench our teeth, hunch our shoulders, and tense our head and neck muscles. These all cause headaches, and some of us can add holding back tears to the list. Those stressors can be relaxed and soothed by smoothing the brow and relieving the pain.

Eye Pillow

MAKES 1 EYE PILLOW

The first time I ever used an eye pillow, it surprised me to find that during headaches or high stress, my eyes responded very well to the gentle weight and the soft, silky material. The weight kept them closed and made me aware of how I was thinking hard and my eyes were moving furiously behind those lids. The weight helps calm that movement. Flaxseed, which are easily found in most grocery stores with a natural section, are the perfect weight and remain cool. Adjust the fragrant herbs to your liking.

1 10-by-10-inch square of silky fabric

1 cup flaxseed

1 tablespoon lavender

1 tablespoon peppermint

1. Fold the fabric in half so the right side is on the inside, and sew one short end and the long side across from the fold.

2. Turn it right-side out.

3. Put the flaxseed, lavender, and peppermint inside.

4. Sew the remaining short end shut.

5. Lie on your back and place the eye pillow across your eyes.

6. Situate the pillow so that the eyes are equally covered by the weight. Relax. Don't be surprised if you fall asleep.

> **Tip:** Migraines can make some people especially sensitive to fragrances, so I also make one with no herbs, just the flaxseed. Can't sew? A closely knit knee-high sock can be filled loosely and tied shut at the end.

Stress Headache Drops
MAKES 2 OUNCES

––––––

The herbs in the blend address pain, tension, and nausea. If possible, recline and close your eyes for 30 minutes. Stress headaches hit me when I don't allow myself to stop and rest. Often, you may need to eat something, or you may be dehydrated. If eyestrain is a part of it, use the Eye Pillow (page 95) while relaxing!

2 tablespoons blue vervain tincture

1 tablespoon valerian tincture

½ tablespoon ginger root tincture

½ tablespoon chamomile tincture

1. In a measuring cup, combine the blue vervain, valerian, ginger root, and chamomile tinctures.

2. Transfer the mixture into a 2-ounce dropper bottle.

3. Label and date the tincture blend.

4. Take 1 dropperful (25 to 30 drops) in 1 ounce of water or juice. Repeat the dose 30 minutes later if needed.

5. Store the tincture blend in a cool, dark place, where it will last for several years.

Settle the Spirit

Stress has a way of taking over. Once it has a grip, it's hard to shake. Stress hormones, harried thoughts, and all the accompanying symptoms and issues collide. Getting them under control and settled is the goal. After that, we can take steps to change the situation if need be.

Soothe-the-Mood Syrup
MAKES ABOUT 10 OUNCES

––––––

These herbs make a beautiful, calming syrup that can be used to sweeten any tea, taken by the spoonful, or blended with tinctures for various other remedies.

CONTINUES →

3 tablespoons rose

3 tablespoons
lemon balm

3 tablespoons
hawthorn berries,
leaves, and flowers

1 cup water

1 cup sugar

½ to ⅓ cup alcohol
of choice

1. In a saucepan over medium-high heat, combine the rose, lemon balm, hawthorn, and water. Bring to a boil.

2. Reduce the heat and bring to a very low simmer for 5 minutes.

3. Turn off the heat and cover the pan, allowing the mixture to steep for 30 minutes or longer.

4. Strain out the liquid (there should be about 6 ounces; if there's less, add a little water).

5. Rinse the pan and return the liquid to the pan.

6. Turn heat to medium.

7. Add the sugar and stir until it is all dissolved.

8. Allow the syrup to reach a boil.

9. Continue cooking for 3 to 4 minutes, skimming off any scum that forms on the surface.

10. Cool and then add the alcohol. Stir to combine.

11. Transfer the syrup to a bottle. Label and date.

12. Store in the refrigerator for up to 6 months.

Skullcap Nerve Tonic
MAKES 4 OUNCES

You get home from work and have dinner plans, but work came home along with you. It was a stressful, upsetting day, and it has left behind the remnants of agitation. If you're having trouble relaxing, try a little tonic.

6 tablespoons skullcap
tincture

2 tablespoons
lavender-infused honey

1. In a bowl, combine the skullcap tincture and lavender-infused honey.

2. Transfer the tonic to a 4-ounce dropper bottle.

3. Label and date the tincture blend.

4. Take 1 to 2 dropperfuls (30 to 50 drops) up to 3 times a day to become centered and present.

5. Store in a cool, dark place, where it will last for several years.

Skin Issues

Stress shows up on the skin in many ways. Rashes, acne, incessant itching, and dry patches can show up as a result of stressed organs, or nervous reactions may cause you to pick at your face or fingers or maybe scratch absentmindedly. It's important to take care of your skin because it is your largest organ, and an infection or serious rash can make you feel miserable. Infections can also lead to more serious medical conditions, so it's best to keep skin healthy in the first place.

Eczema Oil (or Salve)
MAKES 8 OUNCES

It feels so nice to use this blend while it's still warm. The herbs make it a great all-purpose oil that is soothing and healing with properties that fight infection, inflammation, and fungus. It's a good one to keep in your medicine cabinet.

3 tablespoons plantain	3 tablespoons echinacea root
3 tablespoons elderflower	3 tablespoons thyme
	1 cup olive oil

1. Place the plantain, elderflower, echinacea, thyme, and olive oil into a slow cooker and heat to a low simmer.

2. Turn off the heat.

3. Allow oil to cool.

4. Repeat this process 3 times over the next 24 hours.

5. Strain well, pressing as much of the oil from the plant matter as possible.

6. If an oil is desired, transfer to an 8-ounce bottle.

7. Label and date the oil.

8. Store in a cool, dark place. This will keep for about 6 months.

To make the salve

2 tablespoons beeswax pastilles	½ teaspoon colloidal oatmeal or ground baby oatmeal

1. Add the beeswax to ½ cup of the infused oil and heat slowly until the beeswax melts. (I like to start with the oil that has just been strained and is still quite warm. Sometimes no further heat is needed.)

2. Add the oatmeal and mix very well. The oatmeal will cut the greasy feeling, and it's good for the skin.

3. Transfer into small wide-mouth containers. Don't move them or put the lids on until the salve has set.

4. Label and date.

5. If kept cool and dry, salve usually lasts about 6 months.

> **Tip:** To use this most effectively, bathe and lightly dry off. Apply all over to seal in moisture. For feet and hands, apply liberally and cover with socks before climbing into bed.

Hives Spray

MAKES 8 OUNCES

The first time I saw someone develop hives purely from stress and nerves, it was shocking. It was such a clear visual example of how the mind, body, and spirit are intertwined. If you intend to use this spray within a couple of days, it can be stored in the fridge between uses, and there's no need for alcohol preservative. Otherwise, add the alcohol as described.

1¼ cups of water (herbs will absorb some of the water)

¼ cup lemon balm

¼ cup St. John's wort

¼ cup nettle

¼ cup rose

3 tablespoons rubbing alcohol or vodka

1. In a small pot, heat the water to boiling. Once boiling, turn off the heat.

2. Add the lemon balm, St. John's wort, nettle, and rose and steep for about 30 minutes.

3. Strain the mixture through a very fine-mesh strainer and/or cloth (like an old T-shirt).

4. Pour 7 ounces of the liquid into a spray bottle. Add the alcohol.

5. Shake well and use as needed.

6. Store in the refrigerator.

Tip: A tea from these same herbs can be made and taken internally at the same time.

Hives Bath Blend

MAKES ENOUGH FOR 1 BATH

This bath is good for a lot of different things, and hives is one of them. It can soothe chicken pox, poison ivy, sunburn, or prickly heat. My now-grown daughter has always loved baths when she needed a quick de-stress from too much time being social. This is a family favorite!

¼ cup oatmeal

1 tablespoon chamomile

1 tablespoon lavender

1 tablespoon rose petals

1 cup witch hazel

¼ cup baking soda

1. In a muslin bag or gathered into a washcloth closed off with a rubber band, combine the oatmeal, chamomile, lavender, and rose.

2. If cleansing is needed, take a quick shower first.

3. Steep the herb packet in a heatproof pitcher of very hot water while the bath runs.

4. Use tepid or nearly cool water to fill the tub.

5. Add the witch hazel and baking soda and swish to dissolve the baking soda.

6. Pour the tea into the tub and hop in.

7. Relax and let the water soothe the skin.

8. After about 15 minutes, dry off gently without rinsing.

9. Dress in loose clothing made of natural, non-itchy fibers.

Soothe-the-Skin Bath Blend
MAKES ENOUGH FOR 12 BATHS

I started using this after coming in from a day in the garden grimy and uncomfortable from being sweaty and found that it is relaxing, skin soothing, and very pleasant. It's become an herbal blend I keep around at all times. This tub tea can easily be made ahead so it's ready to use when you need it. I use large, heat-sealable tea bags that easily hold ¼ cup of the blend and prepack them all. They stay in a big jar, and all I need to do is grab one and make the tea to dump in the tub!

1 cup plantain	½ cup oatmeal
½ cup rose	¼ cup St. John's wort
½ cup lavender	¼ cup lemon balm

1. In a large bowl, combine the plantain, rose, lavender, oatmeal, St. John's wort, and lemon balm.

2. Transfer to a 1-quart jar.

3. Label and date the bath blend.

4. To use, place ¼ cup into an infuser, muslin bag, large tea bag, washcloth, or whatever you use.

5. Steep the herbs in a heatproof pitcher of very hot water while the bath runs.

6. If cleansing is needed, take a quick shower first.

7. Pour the tea and the packet into the bath.

8. Get in and relax for at least 15 minutes.

9. Dry off gently and dress in loose comfortable clothing (cotton is ideal).

Soothing Bath Vinegar
MAKES ENOUGH FOR 3 BATHS

Vinegar alone is a terrific skin treatment in many situations, several of which can be stress-related. Better yet, vinegar infused with healing herbs can also be a facial toner, an antifungal, and an antibacterial pH-balancing hair and skin "fixer." Once you start using vinegars for bath and body care, you'll find more and more ways to benefit from them.

2 tablespoons plantain	2 tablespoons lavender
2 tablespoons rose	1½ cups apple cider vinegar

1. In a small saucepan over medium-high heat, combine the plantain, rose, lavender, and apple cider vinegar.

2. Bring to a boil and turn off the heat.

3. Cover and steep for about 1 hour.

CONTINUES →

4. Strain well.

5. Transfer to a 12-ounce bottle.

6. Label and date the infused vinegar.

7. Add ½ cup to the bath.

8. Climb in and relax.

> **Note:** Dilute 4 parts water to 1 part infused vinegar to use as a facial toner or hair rinse.

Skin Maintenance

The following recipes are intended to keep your skin healthy so you are better able to fight off the sorts of issues that can result from poor nutrition and lack of rest. Unfortunately, the physical manifestations of chronic and acute stress often show up as disturbances in your skin, hair, and nails.

Custom Bath Blends
MAKES ENOUGH FOR 1 BATH

The following lists will give you some ideas of how to customize recipes for the bath. But you truly cannot go wrong. A nourishing bath can be as simple as adding a single herb with or without some salt. It may turn out that you really enjoy blending baths. If so, there are hundreds of herbs out there that want to be your watery allies! A little research will show you the way.

For normal skin

¼ **cup herb blend (oats, echinacea, chamomile, or lavender)**

¼ **cup milk powder (optional)**

½ **cup Epsom salts (optional)**

For oily skin

¼ **cup herb blend (thyme, sage, peppermint, or rosemary)**

½ **cup baking soda (optional)**

½ **cup Epsom salts (optional)**

For dry skin

¼ **cup herb blend (rose, plantain, chamomile, or oatmeal)**

½ **cup yogurt (optional)**

½ **cup olive oil (optional)**

½ **cup vinegar (optional)**

¼ **cup any kind of powdered milk (optional)**

1 **tablespoon honey (optional)**

1. Choose whatever herbs you have available or would like to use for your skin type.

2. Combine your chosen herbs and make 1 quart of strong infusion from them, steeping for 30 minutes.

3. Add the other ingredients (if using), such as milk, olive oil, baking soda, etc., directly to the tub and mix into the water as it runs.

4. Pour the infusion into the tub.

5. Climb in and relax for at least 15 minutes.

Smooth Skin Salve
MAKES ½ CUP

Stress encourages habits like nail biting, absentminded scratching, and picking at the skin. One of the best ways to avoid infections of hangnails and cuticles is to keep your hands and skin supple, smooth, and healthy. This salve features healing properties of the plantain, the smoothing and soothing rose, and the antibacterial thyme. It is simple and healing.

3 tablespoons thyme-infused olive oil

¼ cup plantain-infused olive oil

3 tablespoons rose-infused olive oil

2 tablespoons beeswax pastilles

1. In a small saucepan over low heat, add the thyme-, rose-, and plantain-infused olive oils.

2. Add the beeswax and gently combine until the beeswax is melted and incorporated.

3. Transfer to 1 or 2 wide-mouthed containers.

4. Label and date the salve.

5. Use as often as needed to keep the hands healthy.

6. Store in a cool, dark place. This will keep for about 6 months.

Sleep

Often we worry about things, relive embarrassing moments, or even go over our saddest experiences when we are trying to go to sleep. Instead of relaxing into sleep, you get more and more anxious and wakeful as your mind loops through an endless array of unwanted thoughts.

Unfortunately, insomnia is an extremely common condition. It can present in any number of ways physically, depending on what kinds of things are keeping you awake. It can range from a cold sweat to just flopping around, unable to get comfortable. There are many ways herbs can help. Some herbal allies include chamomile, lemon balm, and California poppy. Regular exercise and avoiding caffeine can also help you combat stress-induced insomnia.

Relaxing Bath Blend
MAKES ENOUGH FOR 4 BATHS

This bath is great whether or not there's a problem with sleep. Epsom salt is magnesium sulfate, and magnesium is soothing to muscles that might be holding tension. The oats quickly turn the water into a silky treatment for any itch or discomfort, and the rose and lavender both are relaxing and comforting scents in aromatherapy and have skin-soothing properties.

1 cup Epsom salt

¼ cup rose

1 cup oatmeal

¼ cup lavender

CONTINUES →

1. In a bowl, combine the Epsom salt, oatmeal, rose, and lavender.

2. Place a heaping ½ cup of the mixture into the center of a washcloth. Gather the corners of the washcloth and secure with a rubber band, keeping the herbal mixture secure in this bundle.

3. Steep the herb bundle in a heatproof pitcher of very hot water while the bath runs.

4. Pour the contents from the pitcher, including the bundle, into the bath.

5. Keep soap use to a minimum if at all.

Tip: The Snooze-Time Tea Blend (below) tastes great while soaking in this bath. It's an ideal bedtime ritual for you if sleep is hard to come by.

Snooze-Time Tea Blend
MAKES 1 CUP

These two herbs are surprisingly delicious and can be sweetened a bit with honey, if desired. They are also effective at calming; they have rarely let me down, while even being mild and pleasant enough for a young child. Either herb can also be used alone, but each herb works just a little differently. It may be worthwhile to mix up some of this blend and keep it at the ready for a regular nightcap. Even adults benefit from a nighttime routine for ongoing sleep problems, and this blend makes a nice addition.

1 teaspoon chamomile   1 teaspoon lemon balm

1. Choose a mug that feels good in your hands.

2. Put the chamomile and lemon balm into an infuser and place it in the mug.

3. Fill the mug with just-boiled water.

4. The herbs will not become bitter, so they can steep for at least 5 minutes. (The stronger it gets, the better I like it.)

5. Enjoy the warmth of the mug while you sip and drink nightly if desired.

Deep Sleep Drops
MAKES 2 OUNCES

The herbs in this blend combine to soothe and calm the nerves, relax the mind, and stop repetitive thoughts that fail to resolve anything. They promote restful sleep, relieving anxiety, tension, and stress.

2 tablespoons passionflower tincture

2 teaspoons milky oats tincture

2 teaspoons lemon balm tincture

2 teaspoons motherwort tincture

1. In a measuring cup, combine the passionflower, lemon balm, milky oats, and motherwort tinctures.

2. Transfer the mixture into a 2-ounce dropper bottle.

3. Label and date the tincture blend.

4. Take 1 dropperful (25 to 30 drops) in 1 ounce of water 15 to 30 minutes before bed. Repeat the dose 30 minutes later if needed.

5. Store the tincture blend in a cool, dark place, where it will last for several years.

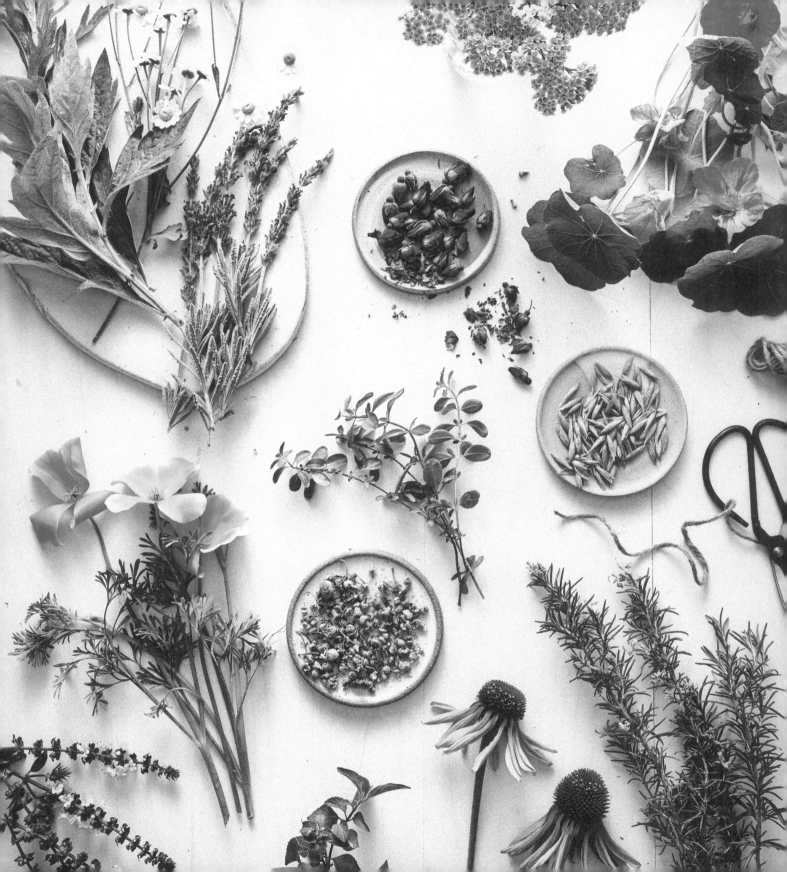

PART THREE

Herbal Allies for Emotional Work

The following 31 herbs were chosen due to their wide-ranging abilities to come to our aid for a variety of issues. Many of them can be grown at home, but all of them are fairly easy to find (sources are provided on page 151). I believe that everyone will find three or four herbs in this selection that they just love and always want to have on hand. These allies will be there for you.

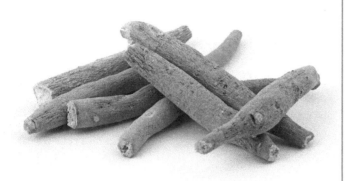

Ashwagandha

LATIN NAME: *Withania somnifera*
ALSO KNOWN NICKNAMES: Indian ginseng, poison gooseberry, winter cherry
FAMILY: Solanaceae

Ashwagandha has long been used in Ayurveda. The West has only started noticing it in the past few decades. Ashwagandha is one of the handful of herbs called *adaptogens*, which means they assist the body in managing stress. Today's world seems to be craving that help, and so ashwagandha is becoming more and more popular. The common name translates as *ashva* = "horse" and *gandha* = "the smell." The root smells like horse sweat. The scent can be easily disguised, though.

QUALITIES: bitter, dry, pungent, warm

THERAPEUTIC ACTIONS: adaptogen, alterative, analgesic, anti-inflammatory, antiseptic, antispasmodic, antitussive, aphrodisiac, anxiolytic, bitter, immuno-modulator, nootropic, sedative, stimulant

IDEAL FOR ADDRESSING: anxiety and stress, depression, fatigue, flagging libido, skin issues, sleep issues, brain fog, general debility

MEDICINAL PARTS USED: While we use the roots for most emotional and energy issues, the leaves, flowers, and seeds are also used in Ayurvedic medicine for various purposes. For instance, poultices of leaves are used to treat boils.

COMMON PREPARATIONS: powder, tincture, capsules

EFFECTIVE APPLICATIONS: The powdered root is traditionally blended with honey and/or ghee (clarified butter) to form a thick paste that is taken a spoonful at a time. This paste can be formed into pills and dried or mixed with warm milk in the evening to help with restlessness to promote sleep. It takes a few days to work, so it may help to combine it with another relaxing herb like passionflower or California poppy for several nights.

Ashwagandha is valuable for people who push themselves to the point of emotional, physical, and mental exhaustion. It supports the adrenals, which this kind of person tends to wear out by constantly pushing that stress button, releasing stress hormones. As an adaptogen, ashwagandha reminds me of the artificial horizon indicator in an airplane. Using a gyroscope, the artificial horizon is steady and true, helping the pilot get back on the right track. Whichever direction is required to level out, ashwagandha will move us in that direction.

RECOMMENDED DOSAGE: 250 to 500 mg daily in capsules long term; tincture: 20 to 60 drops up to 3 times a day

CAUTIONS: Not for use in pregnancy. If on medication for blood pressure, blood sugar, thyroid, or autoimmune issues, check with your physician before using ashwagandha.

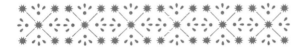

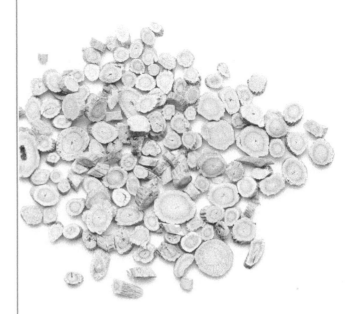

Astragalus

LATIN NAME: *Astragalus membranaceus*
ALSO KNOWN NICKNAMES: *huang qi* (Chinese), milkvetch
FAMILY: Fabaceae

Astragalus is a favorite among herbalists because it can so easily be added to your diet in any kind of soup, stew, infusion, or decoction. It gently supports your health, battles viruses and bacteria, and conditions the way you react to stress. An added bonus is how astragalus promotes a youthful appearance!

QUALITIES: sweet, warm, moist

THERAPEUTIC ACTIONS: adaptogen, supports adrenal function, antiaging, antibacterial, anti-inflammatory, antiviral, diuretic, immune-stimulant, vasodilator

IDEAL FOR ADDRESSING: allergies, diarrhea, fatigue, immune function, mood, stress, upper respiratory infections

MEDICINAL PARTS USED: roots

COMMON PREPARATIONS: soups, teas, extracts, capsules

EFFECTIVE APPLICATIONS: It can be purchased in slices, in powder, or cut and sifted. It is listed (as are many herbs) for everything from hepatitis to diabetes to cancer. For our purposes, we're aiming more at self-limiting illnesses and generally short-term emotional issues.

Astragalus is terrific for preventing colds, flu, and upper respiratory infections as an antiviral that also stimulates the immune system. It's good to have around as part of a tonic that is taken daily during the cold and flu season.

For antiaging, astragalus is used both internally and topically, particularly on the face. The powder can be made into a facial by combining it with mashed fruit, yogurt, or a light oil, or make a cup of tea to drink and another cup to apply to the face.

RECOMMENDED DOSAGE: for typical use, in soup or tea 3 times a day; tincture: 20 to 60 drops up to 3 times a day

CAUTIONS: Can interfere with anti-rejection medication or drugs used to suppress the immune system. Autoimmune diseases could be exacerbated. Safety unknown for pregnancy or breastfeeding.

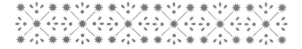

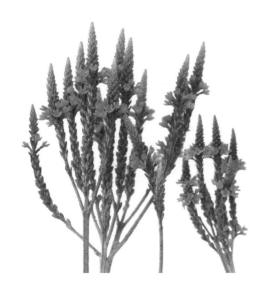

Blue Vervain

LATIN NAME: *Verbena hastata*
ALSO KNOWN NICKNAMES: simpler's joy, holy herb, verbena, vervaine
FAMILY: Verbenaceae

If you've ever seen blue vervain growing, it's plain as day that it's calling to us with the clear blue flowers that look like tiny candles in the meadow. It has been used medicinally in various parts of the world for thousands of years and is known to be one of those herbs that can step in and help at just about any time—meaning it is extremely versatile.

QUALITIES: slightly cooling, drying

THERAPEUTIC ACTIONS: analgesic, anti-spasmodic, bitter, diuretic, expectorant, galactagogue, nervine, relaxant, mild sedative, tonic

IDEAL FOR ADDRESSING: anxiety, chronic bronchitis, depression, digestion, headache, and insomnia kidney stones, milk production, pain, spastic coughing, urinary tract infection

MEDICINAL PARTS USED: aerial parts in flower

COMMON PREPARATIONS: tincture, capsules

EFFECTIVE APPLICATIONS: Blue vervain is specific for neck and shoulder pain, with or without tension headache.

Another way this ally jumps to our assistance is in helping us get to sleep when sore and painful muscles make it tough to drift off. The same is true when coughing won't let you sleep.

RECOMMENDED DOSAGE: tincture: 25 drops 2 or 3 times a day; capsules or pills: follow label instructions; tea is very bitter, so it's difficult to drink too much, but 3 cups a day is a good guideline

CAUTIONS: Large doses can result in upset stomach and vomiting. Avoid if kidney disease is present.

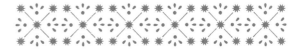

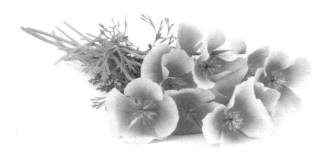

California Poppy

LATIN NAME: *Eschscholzia californica*
ALSO KNOWN NICKNAME: cup of gold
FAMILY: Papaveraceae

This state flower of California is a beautiful yellow and orange (sometimes pinks as well) poppy. Often the seeds are part of wildflower mixes and grow easily into an unassuming little beauty that is a non-addictive narcotic that contains no opiates. This pain-relieving sleep aid deserves a place in your home apothecary.

QUALITIES: cool, dry, bitter

THERAPEUTIC ACTIONS: mildly analgesic, antispasmodic, anxiolytic, hypnotic, nervine, sedative

IDEAL FOR ADDRESSING: insomnia, aches, chronic pain, headaches, nervous agitation, bedwetting in children, anxiety

MEDICINAL PARTS USED: whole plant, root-flowering tops

COMMON PREPARATIONS: tincture, tea, capsules

EFFECTIVE APPLICATIONS: California poppy is a dream come true for those suffering from jerking limbs and restless legs that repeatedly awaken them or disturb their sleep. Sometimes people aren't aware of how often they become almost awake during the night, but if they sleep with a partner, *they* know! A dropperful of tincture before bed can help everyone reach a deeper level of sleep.

The tea is a nice assist for overtired, overwhelmed, cranky, verge-of-a-headache times.

It can be helpful for both PTSD and withdrawal from opiate drugs—both under the direction of professionals.

RECOMMENDED DOSAGE: 20 to 30 drops of the tincture before bed and repeat after 30 minutes if needed; tea can be drunk as needed (it can be bitter, especially with a long brew, so most people won't overdo it)

CAUTIONS: Do not combine with medications for sleep, sedation, or anxiety. Avoid in pregnancy and breastfeeding. Don't drive or operate machinery.

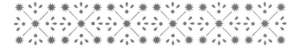

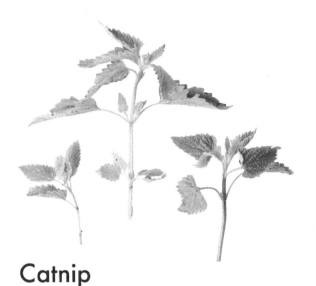

Catnip

LATIN NAME: *Nepeta cataria*
ALSO KNOWN NICKNAMES: catmint, catswort, cat nep, field balm, nep, herb catta
FAMILY: Lamiaceae

While catnip owes its name to its stimulant effect on cats, it affects humans very differently. Before tea (*Camilla sinensis*) became available to most parts of the world, catnip tea was routinely served as a beverage. The component nepetalactone is responsible for most of the actions of the herb, and in recent years it has been researched in treatment of everything from ADHD to MRSA to cancer. In the meantime, we know that it will help with several issues like flatulence or relaxation.

QUALITIES: cool, dry, and slightly bitter

THERAPEUTIC ACTIONS: mildly anesthetic, antibiotic, antispasmodic, diaphoretic, immune-stimulating, nervine, relaxing, sedative

IDEAL FOR ADDRESSING: lack of appetite, constipation, gas, colic in babies, intestinal cramps, indigestion, lack of menstruation

MEDICINAL PARTS USED: leaves and flowers prior to bloom for teas, tincture, vinegar, or any kind of internal application; best while in bloom if insect-repellent properties are desired

COMMON PREPARATIONS: tea, tincture, vinegar

EFFECTIVE APPLICATIONS: A cup of tea or a dose of tincture can settle down many of the digestive problems brought on by emotional issues, such as cramping and excess gas. Catnip is mild enough to help an overexcited child relax. The essential oil of catnip is a very good mosquito repellant. Essential oil is present in the leaves and flowers of the plants, so rub the undersides (especially) of the leaves and the flowers on skin to shoo away skeeters.

RECOMMENDED DOSAGE: most often used as a tea 1 to 3 cups a day; tincture: 20 to 30 drops 2 to 4 times a day

CAUTIONS: Very large doses may cause vomiting. Avoid catnip while pregnant or if there are kidney or liver issues.

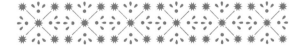

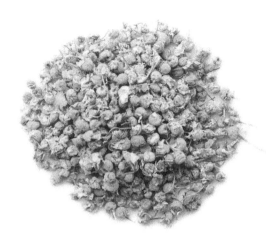

Chamomile

LATIN NAME: *Matricaria recutita* (German); *Chamaemelum nobile* (Roman)
ALSO KNOWN NICKNAMES: chamomile, mayweed, earth apple, mantazilla
FAMILY: Asteraceae

This lightly apple-scented herb lives up to the name *Matricaria*. I believe that has the connotation of "mother," and in Latin, one meaning of *matrix* is womb. Chamomile is gentle and seems to be able to fix almost anything, just like a mother would. Certainly Peter Rabbit's mother knew that it would help with her naughty little bunny's tummy ache and restlessness.

There are some slight differences between German and Roman chamomiles, but they are more pronounced in aromatherapy. For our purposes, they can be used interchangeably.

QUALITIES: slightly bitter, slightly warming, relaxing

THERAPEUTIC ACTIONS: anti-allergenic, antibacterial, anti-inflammatory, carminative, sedative

IDEAL FOR ADDRESSING: anxiety, gastrointestinal disorders, inflammation, insomnia, menstrual disorders, muscle spasms, overtired, restlessness, soothing skin, upset stomach, ulcers, wounds

MEDICINAL PARTS USED: flowers

COMMON PREPARATIONS: tea, sachets, tincture

EFFECTIVE APPLICATIONS: I have used very warm tea bags to soothe eye sties, which are staph infections of the eyelids. Having caught them early, I've been a little shocked that they did not progress and by the next day were gone. Chamomile is a delightful remedy for indigestion and cramps by helping to reduce gas. It calms and relaxes while soothing inflammation in the lower digestive tract and bowel, making it useful for irritable bowel syndrome. Try a cup of tea after a meal.

RECOMMENDED DOSAGE: 2 to 3 cups of tea a day; tincture: 40 to 60 drops 3 times a day or as needed; barring an allergy, chamomile is very safe

CAUTIONS: People who have allergies to plants in the aster family may have a problem with chamomile.

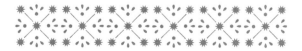

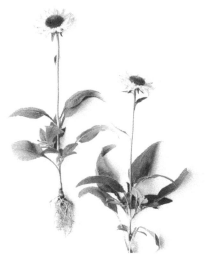

Echinacea

LATIN NAME: *E. angustifolia* and *E. purpurea* most often

ALSO KNOWN NICKNAMES: purple coneflower, snakeroot, black sampson, red sunflower, Indian head

FAMILY: Asteraceae

Echinacea has been a subject of debate for the past 15 or 20 years, and although science may never be able to come to an agreement on whether it is effective, herbalists have plenty of anecdotal experience, and know that it does in fact have many wonderful benefits for us.

QUALITIES: bitter, cool, dry

THERAPEUTIC ACTIONS: analgesic, antibacterial, antifungal, anti-inflammatory, antioxidant, antiseptic, antiviral, astringent, stimulates and supports the immune system, tonic, vulnerary

IDEAL FOR ADDRESSING: anxiety, headache, inflammation, colds and flu, pain, skin issues

MEDICINAL PARTS USED: all parts of the plant are medicinal—root to flower

COMMON PREPARATIONS: tincture, tea, capsules

EFFECTIVE APPLICATIONS: When illness starts going around the office, pull out the echinacea. It's best not to take it as a daily tonic kind of preventive, but it's good when there's a threat. Follow a 2-weeks-on, 1-week-off pulse.

Try rinsing teen skin with echinacea tea when acne is acting up.

RECOMMENDED DOSAGE: 3 to 4 cups of tea a day; tincture: 40 to 60 drops up to 4 times a day; capsules: follow directions on label; best to take echinacea by pulsing, which means to take for 2 weeks (or days) and then not for 1 week (or day)

CAUTIONS: Some people are allergic to it, so use caution if there are other known plant allergies. Large, frequent doses can cause nausea. Some people don't need to take large doses for this side effect to occur. Avoid in the case of autoimmune disease.

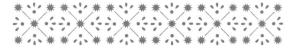

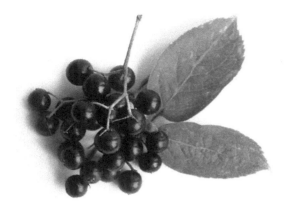

Elderberry and Elderflower

LATIN NAME: *Sambucus nigra, Sambucus cerulean, Sambucus canadensis*

ALSO KNOWN NICKNAMES: elder, elderberry, black elder, European elder, European elderberry and European black elderberry, Mexican Elderberry. Blossoms are sometimes referred to as "elder blow"

FAMILY: Adoxaceae

Pharmaceutical labs can't always forecast the correct strain of flu for which to make a vaccine, but luckily, elderberry can handle them all.

QUALITIES: bitter, drying, cool, slightly sweet

THERAPEUTIC ACTIONS: alterative, anti-inflammatory, antioxidant, antiviral, astringent, demulcent, diuretic, emollient, expectorant, immune-enhancing, laxative

IDEAL FOR ADDRESSING: viral infections (cold and flu), joint pain, edema, constipation

MEDICINAL PARTS USED: flowers, berries; leaves for external use only

COMMON PREPARATIONS: tea, tincture, syrup, cough drops, gummies, jelly, juice, vinegar

EFFECTIVE APPLICATIONS: I usually use juice. To make it using fresh berries, add just enough water to a pan full of berries so that they don't scorch before bursting and releasing juice. For dry berries, add an amount of water equal in volume to the berries. Strain very well. When cool, freeze it in ¼-inch sheets in baggies. Break off what you need.

For colds, elderflower blossoms are traditionally blended with mint and another herb called yarrow with great success.

RECOMMENDED DOSAGE: flexible; berry juice, syrup, tincture, or tea to stop illness after exposure: 4 times a day for at least 3 days; as a daily preventive, 25 drops a day; flower tea or tincture 3 or 4 times a day

CAUTIONS: The berries and flowers are safe for use, but the leaves and twigs are toxic. Large amounts of raw berries may cause stomach distress. The leaves are sometimes used to make a salve or oil for bumps and bruises. Excessive use of berries or flowers can cause diarrhea.

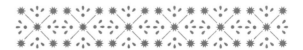

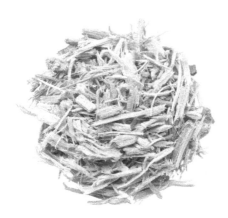

Eleuthero

LATIN NAME: *Eleutherococcus senticosus*
ALSO KNOWN NICKNAMES: eleuthero, Siberian ginseng
FAMILY: Araliaceae

Eleuthero was the first adaptogen I ever worked with. At the time it generally went by the name Siberian ginseng, and it has been an amazing ally for me. It is not a true ginseng (Panax), but because it has so many common properties as an adaptogen, it got the nickname. To lessen confusion, the US government in 2002 ruled that it be called "eleuthero." Research was conducted using factory workers in big, windowless buildings in Siberia. Compared to the control group, those taking the eleuthero improved in every measureable way—productivity, mental alertness, stamina, sick days, job satisfaction, and so on.

Be sure to use reputable sources for eleuthero (see Resources, page 151) because it is often adulterated.

QUALITIES: warming, pungent

THERAPEUTIC ACTIONS: adaptogen, adrenal tonic, anticancer, antidiabetic, antiviral, immune-stimulating, neuroprotective, tonic

IDEAL FOR ADDRESSING: anxiety, brain function, cold, fatigue, flu, herpes, stress

MEDICINAL PARTS USED: root mostly; less often, leaves

COMMON PREPARATIONS: tincture, capsules, tablets, tea, powder

EFFECTIVE APPLICATIONS: For fatigue and a dread of the daily grind, try taking eleuthero for a month. Stop for a week and then take for another month. Evaluate from there. Eleuthero can be helpful for tackling big or super-boring tasks, providing stamina and the ability to stay on task.

RECOMMENDED DOSAGE: tincture: 30 to 50 drops 1 to 3 times a day; follow label instructions for capsules

CAUTIONS: Although side effects are rare, eleuthero should be avoided in high doses by individuals with very high blood pressure, insomnia, irritability, melancholy, and anxiety.

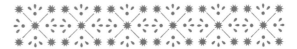

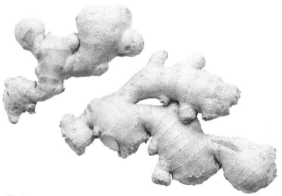

Ginger

LATIN NAME: *Zingiber officinale*
ALSO KNOWN NICKNAMES: ginger root, awapuhi
FAMILY: Zingiberaceae

Most of us first experienced this pungent and aromatically delicious root in the soft drink ginger ale, perhaps while we were sick as a child. It really is a miracle for nausea of all kinds. If there was nothing else this beautiful plant had to offer, that would be enough. Of course, there's much more. In fact, research is ongoing, and we are just scratching the surface of all the benefits this spicy, hot root has to offer.

QUALITIES: pungent, hot, sweet

THERAPEUTIC ACTIONS: analgesic, anti-inflammatory, antibacterial, antifungal, antiviral, carminative, diaphoretic, immune boosting, neuroprotective, thermogenic, thins blood

IDEAL FOR ADDRESSING: arthritis, colds, flu, gas, indigestion, inflammation, morning sickness, general nausea, motion sickness, externally and internally for joint pain, migraines

MEDICINAL PARTS USED: root

COMMON PREPARATIONS: tea, tincture, bath, crystallized, fresh, pickled, powdered, syrup

EFFECTIVE APPLICATIONS: Ginger potentiates other herbal preparations, so I add some to almost any medicinal herb tea. My favorite cold and flu tea is sage, lemon, honey, and lots of grated fresh ginger.

Crystallized or candied ginger is a must for first aid kits and glove compartments. It addresses car and motion sickness in a snap.

RECOMMENDED DOSAGE: tea is spicy, so 3 mugs a day is plenty; tincture: 25 to 50 drops a few times a day

CAUTIONS: Ginger thins the blood, so if you are on anticoagulant medicines, use in moderation. More than 1 teaspoon powder or 1 tablespoon fresh may cause heartburn.

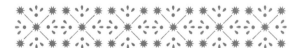

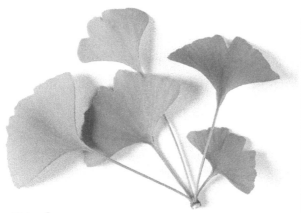

Ginkgo

LATIN NAME: *Ginkgo biloba*
ALSO KNOWN NICKNAMES: maidenhair
FAMILY: Ginkgoaceae

The ginkgo tree in autumn has a specific clear yellow leaf. If you learn that color, you can identify a tree in a wooded area from 50 yards. The fruit of the trees contains edible seeds, but the outer flesh can cause contact dermatitis and smells horrible.

This native of China is thought to be more than 270 million years old as a species and is considered a living fossil. There are trees much older than 1,000 years old. Interestingly, these old trees show no sign of aging, as they continue to put out shoots and leaves and remain strong. Certainly, they have something to teach us. Ginkgo is being studied for brain health, eye health, and various other issues that involve circulation.

QUALITIES: sweet, sour, bitter, neutral

THERAPEUTIC ACTIONS: analgesic, anti-inflammatory, anxiolytic, circulatory stimulant, hypotensive, nootropic

IDEAL FOR ADDRESSING: circulation problems, memory loss, Alzheimer's disease symptoms, glaucoma, vertigo, tinnitus, hearing loss, sexual dysfunction

MEDICINAL PARTS USED: leaves mostly; nuts in some parts of the world

COMMON PREPARATIONS: tincture, capsules, pills

EFFECTIVE APPLICATIONS: People always say, "If I could remember, I'd take ginkgo every day." It is believed to improve blood flow throughout the brain, including the small capillaries, etc., so that the brain is healthier and oxygenated. That ability to increase circulation is the main function that is behind the maladies that ginkgo addresses.

RECOMMENDED DOSAGE: tincture: 25 to 50 drops 3 times a day for 2 months and then evaluate; capsules or pills: follow directions on label

CAUTIONS: May interact with blood-thinning medications such as Coumadin (Warfarin) and aspirin. It may also interact with medications for high blood pressure and diabetes, so check with your doctor before taking ginkgo.

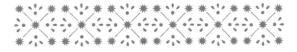

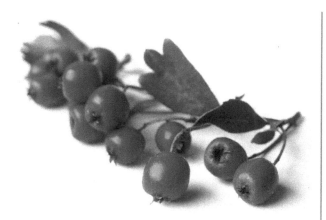

Hawthorn

LATIN NAME: *Crataegus laevigata*

ALSO KNOWN NICKNAMES: English hawthorn, maybush, may tree, haw, quickset, thornapple, whitethorn, cockspur, cockspur thorn, Washington thorn, red haw, summer haw

FAMILY: Roseaceae

A very popular and storied tree, hawthorn has a long history of use for protecting and supporting the heart muscle. This is one of those things, though, where it is essential to get a good, clear diagnosis before embarking on self-care. We all, but particularly women, too often overlook symptoms until it's too late. Hawthorn will be there when it's time to support or heal.

QUALITIES: warming, sour, slightly sweet

THERAPEUTIC ACTIONS: anxiolytic, antihypertensive, anti-inflammatory, antioxidant, astringent, cardiotonic, carminative, diuretic, relaxant

IDEAL FOR ADDRESSING: anxiety, high blood pressure, heart failure, heart tonic, poor digestion, heartbreak, stress

MEDICINAL PARTS USED: berry, leaves, flowers

COMMON PREPARATIONS: tincture, tea, capsules, pills

EFFECTIVE APPLICATIONS: During heartbreak or grief, there can be pain or a feeling of constriction. Please have it checked to be safe. Hawthorn is the herb to help this pain. Many herbalists add hawthorn to their elixirs for heartbreak. Hawthorn also is useful in restless anxiety.

RECOMMENDED DOSAGE: dosage depends on the ailment; for prevention, tincture: 20 to 30 drops 3 times a day; capsules and pills: follow directions on label

CAUTIONS: If taking heart medications, check with your doctor before using hawthorn because it can interfere with or increase their effectiveness.

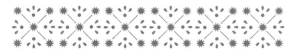

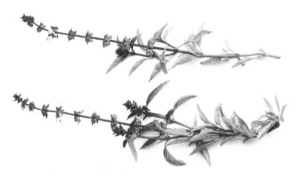

Holy Basil

LATIN NAME: *Ocimum tenuiflorum*
ALSO KNOWN NICKNAMES: Tulsi, Tulasi, *Ocimum sanctum*, Indian basil, "the incomparable one," hot basil, "queen of herbs," sacred basil
FAMILY: Lamiaceae

Holy basil has this wild ability to let you stand off to the side, objectively look at a situation, and change perspective. It is an herb to get to know. In Hindu culture, the plant in so important and so revered that there are special planters built in the central courtyards that contain holy basil. The woody stems are cut, carved into beads, and used in prayer malas.

It is that special. The Hindu people believe the plant is a deity; that the goddess Lakshmi resides within. It's no wonder, really. In addition to the really amazing emotional rewards it offers, it has been used for everything from toothaches to malaria, with varying levels of success.

QUALITIES: both hot and cooling; also both pungent and sweet

THERAPEUTIC ACTIONS: adaptogen, analgesic, antibacterial, antidepressant, antifungal, anti-inflammatory, antioxidant, antiviral, anxiolytic, balances chakras, diuretic, expectorant, grounding, clears negatives, nervine, neuroprotective, supports immune system, tonic

IDEAL FOR ADDRESSING: stress, ulcers, joint pain, headache, cold, flu, toothache, skin issues, inflammation

MEDICINAL PARTS USED: aerial parts of the plant

COMMON PREPARATIONS: tea, tincture, pills, capsules

EFFECTIVE APPLICATIONS: Using holy basil and elderberry (with extensive handwashing and not touching doorknobs or handles), I managed to stay healthy for 3 years when caring for an immune-compromised person.

Holy basil can give you courage for facing things like auditions, tests, unpleasant confrontations, and negative people.

RECOMMENDED DOSAGE: tincture: 25 to 50 drops 3 or 4 times a day; 4 cups of tea a day; pills and capsules: follow label directions

CAUTIONS: *May* lower fertility during use.

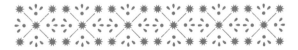

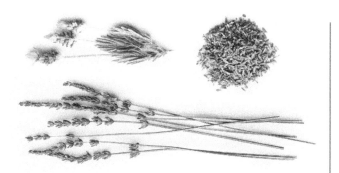

Lavender

LATIN NAME: *Lavandula officinalis* or *Lavender spp.*

ALSO KNOWN NICKNAMES: lavandula, common, English, French, garden, spike, sweet, and true lavender

FAMILY: Lamiaceae

Before becoming familiar with lavender, I'd read odes to her beauty, raves about the fragrance, and, of course, unbelievable praise for her benefits. The first sniff of lavender essential oil was a disappointment because it is fairly medicinal instead of the floral nirvana I was expecting. When using lavender buds in tea or cooking, that medicinal flavor and scent can quickly overwhelm other flavors, so always use it sparingly. The relaxing properties of lavender are renowned and well deserved.

QUALITIES: cool and warm, stimulating and relaxing, pungent and bitter

THERAPEUTIC ACTIONS: antibiotic, antidepressant, antifungal, anti-inflammatory, antiseptic, antispasmodic, antiviral, aromatic, carminative, hepatic, relaxant, sedative

IDEAL FOR ADDRESSING: anxiety, bloating, burns, depression, fungal infection, headache, insomnia, intestinal gas, nausea, skin issues, stress, sunburn, upset stomach

MEDICINAL PARTS USED: flowers, although all aerial parts are potent

COMMON PREPARATIONS: tea, rarely tincture, capsules, bath tea, vinegar

EFFECTIVE APPLICATIONS: Try infusing some olive oil with lavender. It's excellent to massage into sore muscles or on the temples for headaches or as a massage oil to relax. A small amount could also be added to the bath.

A cup of mint tea with a pinch of lavender is great for relaxation or nausea. For tea, it is usually used as a part of a blend because it isn't pleasant alone.

RECOMMENDED DOSAGE: tea: drink as often as needed; tincture: 20 to 30 drops as needed; capsules: as listed on label

CAUTIONS: There have been overblown reports of lavender causing prepubertal gynecomastia in boys (though no mention in girls that I'm aware of, and only three boys specifically) that refer to the essential oil, and we are talking about much less concentrated preparations.

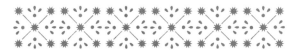

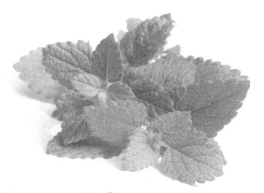

Lemon Balm

LATIN NAME: *Melissa officinalis*
ALSO KNOWN NICKNAMES: lemon balm, melissa balm, bee balm, sweet balm, honey plant, English balm
FAMILY: Lamiaceae

Lemon balm is a great plant to grow, and unfortunately it is much better either fresh or freshly dried than it is possible to purchase. It is sometimes called the "lemon pledge plant" because it smells like the furniture polish. Even though the scent is very strong, it fades along with the flavor within a few months of drying.

Ask five people what they love most about lemon balm, and you'll get five different answers. One person will say it is their go-to for colds, and another will love the way it calms anxiety. Still another will talk about insomnia, and so on. Even when the fragrance has faded, lemon balm will continue to calm, heal, and soothe.

QUALITIES: cold, dry, slightly bitter

THERAPEUTIC ACTIONS: antidepressant, antispasmodic, antiviral, antioxidant, carminative, nervine, nootropic, sedative

IDEAL FOR ADDRESSING: anxiety, cognitive function, cold sores, cramps, headaches, herpes, indigestion, insomnia, mood, nausea, nerve pain, seasonal affective disorder, shingles, stress

MEDICINAL PARTS USED: leaves, best before flowering

COMMON PREPARATIONS: tea, tincture, glycerite, vinegar, infused oil, salve, hydrosol, powder

EFFECTIVE APPLICATIONS: Due to strong antiviral properties, lemon balm is effective on various herpes rashes, like cold sores, chicken pox, shingles, and genital herpes. I love the hydrosol personally (but I have a distiller, so it's easy for me to get), but a strong infusion in a spray bottle is very good, too.

Stress have you unable to think straight? Have some lemon balm and relax.

RECOMMENDED DOSAGE: tincture: 40 to 60 drops 3 to 4 times daily as needed; tea: as needed; capsules or pills: as listed on label; use topically as needed

CAUTIONS: Avoid internal use if using thyroid medication, as it will interfere.

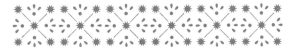

Marshmallow Root

LATIN NAME: *Althaea officinalis*
ALSO KNOWN NICKNAMES: mallards, cheeses, mallow, white mallow, common marshmallow, mortification root, sweet weed
FAMILY: Malvaceae

Up until about 100 years ago, marshmallow root was cooked down and sweetened, and eventually gelatin was added to help it dry out more quickly since it was such a popular confection the shops couldn't keep up. Medicinally, marshmallow was being used thousands of years earlier for healing wounds and sore throats. There's a long history where marshmallow was tried for many different maladies. It falls in and out of favor, but it is always waiting for us.

QUALITIES: sweet, cooling, moistening

THERAPEUTIC ACTIONS: anti-inflammatory, antispasmodic, antitussive, demulcent, diuretic, emollient, nervine, relaxant, tonic, vulnerary

IDEAL FOR ADDRESSING: bronchitis, burns, constipation, dry cough, diarrhea, heartburn, reflux, skin irritation, sore throat, stomach, urinary tract inflammation, ulcerative colitis, ulcers

MEDICINAL PARTS USED: mainly root; also flowers and leaves

COMMON PREPARATIONS: capsules, cream, lotion, tea, tincture, syrup, dried, poultices

EFFECTIVE APPLICATIONS: The very slippery, soothing mucilage that is created with marshmallow and liquid is perfect for soothing mucus membranes all the way from the mouth to the anus. Infuse it in cool or room-temperature water overnight, and drink the thick, soothing beverage in the morning. If the texture is an issue, whip it up in the blender with a few other things—like banana, yogurt, and so on.

A poultice of marshmallow applied to chapped, irritated skin is very healing and soothing.

RECOMMENDED DOSAGE: follow label directions on purchased products

CAUTIONS: Drink a full glass of water (or tea) when taking marshmallow. It may interfere with some medications, particularly those treating blood sugar. Wait an hour between taking marshmallow and taking other medications.

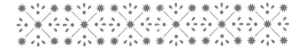

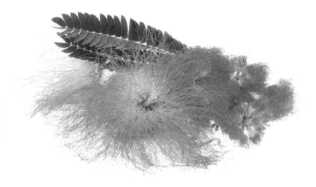

Mimosa

LATIN NAME: *Albizia julibrissin*
ALSO KNOWN NICKNAMES: Tree of Happiness, silk tree, albizzia
FAMILY: Leguminosae

The beautiful, fragrant pink flowers resemble puffs of tiny fiber optic wires, and they glow from within. The leaves are sensitive and fold up when touched. When we look at plants and ask them what they have to offer us, mimosa is very clear. It brings back the light in our hearts and protects us from that which hurts us. It's striking, really. Rarely is it so easy to see the ally and the offer. In a storm, the tree sheds branches, as if to say, "Here, take my bark to protect you from the storm." If this tree grows near you, don't pass it up because it is very special.

QUALITIES: cooling, moistening

THERAPEUTIC ACTIONS: flowers: carminative, digestive, sedative, tonic, cheering, lightening; bark: anodyne, carminative, diuretic, grounding, sedative, stimulant, tonic, vermifuge, vulnerary

IDEAL FOR ADDRESSING: anxiety, depression, grief, sleep problems (insomnia), sore throat, blue or unstable moods, swelling associated with trauma

MEDICINAL PARTS USED: bark and flowers

COMMON PREPARATIONS: tea, tincture, capsules

EFFECTIVE APPLICATIONS: I use a combination that is heavy on bark, light on flowers. The flowers are too "spacey" alone, and I'm a person who needs to be anchored (bark). There is nothing I've found like the combination of mimosa and holy basil for easing the kind of intense, intractable sadness that has a presence of its own. The two together reminds you that tomorrow is another day.

Anxiety responds beautifully to the bark-heavy tincture or decoction.

RECOMMENDED DOSAGE: tincture: 40 to 80 drops up to 3 times daily as needed; tea: 3 or 4 times a day; capsules: as noted on label

CAUTIONS: Not recommended during pregnancy.

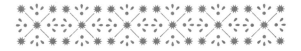

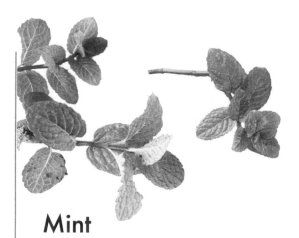

Mint

LATIN NAME: *Mentha spp.*
ALSO KNOWN NICKNAMES: meadow tea
FAMILY: Lamiaceae

Mint grows wild around streams and meadows around here, so children who used to wander freely knew the plant and brought it home to make tea. It is a flavoring in all kinds of candy and ice cream and is sometimes used in savory dishes. Meadow tea is a spearmint (of which there are many), and the mild, soothing, and cooling flavor is something we all recognize. Peppermint, with a higher menthol content, is often used medicinally.

QUALITIES: cooling

THERAPEUTIC ACTIONS: antibacterial, antifungal, antihistamine, anti-inflammatory, antioxidant, anxiolytic, carminative, refrigerant

IDEAL FOR ADDRESSING: anxiety, congestion, coughs, cramps, fatigue, gas, indigestion, nausea, stress

MEDICINAL PARTS USED: leaves before bloom

COMMON PREPARATIONS: tea, tincture, bath tea, candy, gum, syrup

EFFECTIVE APPLICATIONS: A foot soak using peppermint is a great pick-me-up after a long day on your feet and will help get rid of any foot fungus. Increase the antifungal activity by using apple cider vinegar as the liquid.

A cup of spearmint tea after dinner helps digestion and may just help with fatigue.

A good cup of peppermint tea makes a head full of congestion feel better. Breathe in the steam while drinking.

RECOMMENDED DOSAGE: tea: can be drunk as desired; tincture or syrup: as needed; mints are very safe, so use as desired

CAUTIONS: Peppermint can *increase* heartburn or reflux while spearmint *helps*. Note: We are *not* talking about the essential oil of mint here, as that is very concentrated and has completely different instructions. Much of the information out there is about the essential oil, and some recommend internal use. Essential oils should only be taken internally at the direction of certified aromatherapists.

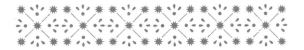

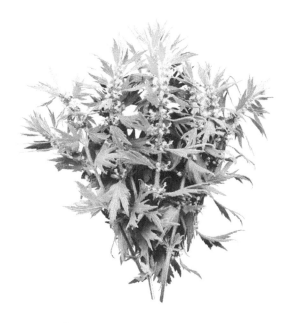

Motherwort

LATIN NAME: *Leonurus cardiaca*
ALSO KNOWN NICKNAMES: lion's tail, lionheart, mother's herb, mother's little helper
FAMILY: Lamiaceae

Thinking about motherwort usually makes me smile because my calmest, most level-headed friend told me she uses it when the kids are on her last nerve, and I just can't picture what they did to get there. The plant is quite distinctive. The young leaves are busy, with lots of lobes and crinkles. As the plant ages, the upper leaves often are three-lobed and remind me of dinosaur footprints. I'm pretty sure if you see them, you'll agree (or just roll your eyes like my family). The flowers grow in spikes like others in the mint family, but be careful—they're prickly!

QUALITIES: cool, bitter, dry, stimulating

THERAPEUTIC ACTIONS: analgesic, antibacterial, antifungal, antioxidant, antispasmodic, astringent, cardiotonic, circulatory stimulant, diaphoretic, diuretic, emmenagogue, immune stimulant, laxative, nervine, sedative, tonic, uterine tonic, vasodilator

IDEAL FOR ADDRESSING: anxiety, rapid or irregular heartbeat, headaches, irritability, melancholy, menopause symptoms, menstrual cramping, mood swings, PMS, sadness, uterine issues

MEDICINAL PARTS USED: flowering 6- to 8-inch tops, leaves, stem, and flowers

COMMON PREPARATIONS: tincture, capsules, occasionally tea

EFFECTIVE APPLICATIONS: Motherwort tincture can really help with hot flashes and night sweats. Most of the women I know agree that hot flashes come along when something shakes them up. It can be almost unnoticeable. It makes sense that motherwort helps those. Motherwort is also stunning for PMS, and for the irritability, discomfort, bloating and cramps, it's a blessing.

RECOMMENDED DOSAGE: tincture: 20 to 30 drops 3 times a day; capsules: follow label directions; in tea, the bitterness will limit use

CAUTIONS: Clear with your doctor if you are on heart medications. Should not be used during pregnancy or early in the process of menopause (while menstruation is still taking place—although irregularly).

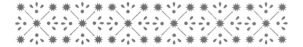

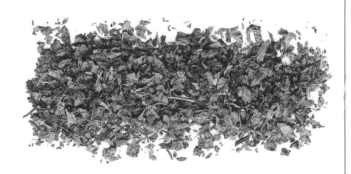

Nettle

LATIN NAME: *Urtica dioica*

ALSO KNOWN NICKNAMES: nettles, burn hazel

FAMILY: Lamiaceae

It is unusual for all parts of a plant to be useful, but that is the case with nettle. The roots are best known as support for aging prostates. The leaves are food and medicine and what we'll discuss here. The seeds are energizing. The stems are worked similarly to flax stalks and make a sturdy fiber or cordage. It is found around the world and grows and spreads with wild abandon. This is one of the plants that we need to get to know and work with in order to stop using such damaging farming practices. People with severe arthritis or gout intentionally "sting" their joint, and find that it relieves inflammation. And if that weren't enough, I planted it by my back door and now have a botanical burglar alarm.

QUALITIES: drying, heating, sweet, salty

MEDICINAL PARTS USED: leaves before bloom, roots, seeds

THERAPEUTIC ACTIONS: antibacterial, antihistamine, anti-inflammatory, astringent, decongestant, diuretic, expectorant, nutritive, styptic, tonic

IDEAL FOR ADDRESSING: allergies, anemia, cramping, eczema, edema, fatigue, gout, hot flashes, water retention, general weakness

COMMON PREPARATIONS: tea, tincture, capsules, foods, bath tea

EFFECTIVE APPLICATIONS: In the spring, my family eats a lot of nettles as a vegetable. It comes up very early in the spring, and just moving around some leaves exposes all we need. There is almost nothing better than a big plate of steamed and buttered nettles. It's one of those dishes that you can feel nourishing you as you eat. It's a great energy builder. For seasonal allergies, we have lots of nettle infusions with local bee pollen.

RECOMMENDED DOSAGE: as desired

CAUTIONS: As this is an herb that can flush out toxins, etc., be sure to stay hydrated, and add some plantain or marshmallow powder to infusions.

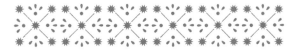

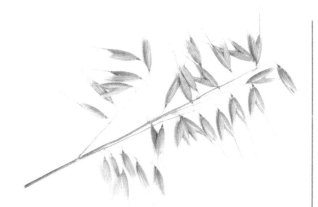

Oats

LATIN NAME: *Avena sativa*

ALSO KNOWN NICKNAMES: wild oats, common oats, milky oats, oatstraw

FAMILY: Poaceae

Avena sativa is a plant that can nourish in almost every stage of growth. The immature grain in the milky stage is very much sought after; the stems, or straw, are extremely nourishing to the nerves; and finally there are oats, which we usually make into breakfast or cookies without recognizing that they too are amazing medicine for us.

QUALITIES: moist, sweet, warming

THERAPEUTIC ACTIONS: antidepressant, nervine, nutritive, restorative

IDEAL FOR ADDRESSING: adrenal exhaustion, anxiety, baby blues, difficulty concentrating, depression, fatigue, gout, irregularity, loss of libido, nervous tension, obesity, skin, stress

MEDICINAL PARTS USED: all aerial parts

COMMON PREPARATIONS: tincture, tea, foods, bath tea

EFFECTIVE APPLICATIONS: Eating oatmeal helps with irregularity, and it is thought that some people who eat it daily lose weight since the oatmeal makes them feel full longer.

Oatstraw and milky oats are an incredible tonic for the nerves, supporting and strengthening them gradually while also having a more immediate relaxing and soothing effect.

RECOMMENDED DOSAGE: As desired. All forms of the plant and their formulations are fine to use in larger doses (or servings) than typical herbs. Teas are often made into very concentrated infusions, although they can also easily be part of a blend; tincture: 4 or 5 dropperfuls 3 times a day

CAUTIONS: Oats are pretty safe!

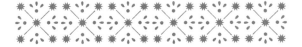

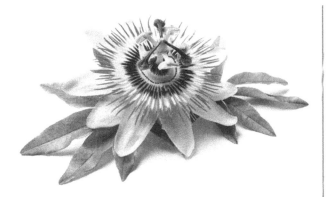

Passionflower

LATIN NAME: *Passiflora incarnata*
ALSO KNOWN NICKNAMES: maypop, passion vine, apricot vine
FAMILY: Passifloraceae

Passionflower is a simply stunning flower, and if it is growing where it is hardy, the vine is vigorous, can be invasive, and wraps around anything that gets in its way. All along the vine are curly tendrils. When I harvest passionflower for tincture or tea, I make sure to get lots of the tendrils in the mix. Using the doctrine of signatures, which means that the plant tells us what it is for with its appearance, the tendrils make me think of how this herb is used for helping to stop circular thinking, so into the mix they go!

QUALITIES: cooling, drying

THERAPEUTIC ACTIONS: analgesic, anxiolytic, antidepressant, antispasmodic, hypnotic, hypotensive, nervine

IDEAL FOR ADDRESSING: addiction withdrawal, anxiety, busy brain, muscle spasms, nerve pain, shingles, sleeplessness

MEDICINAL PARTS USED: leaves, stems, flowers

COMMON PREPARATIONS: tea, tincture, capsules, pills

EFFECTIVE APPLICATIONS: Passionflower tea or tincture relaxes in several different ways. It is best known for stopping circular thinking, or when the brain goes over and over the same (usually unpleasant) thoughts. It is a hypnotic herb, meaning that it is quite strong, and it also relaxes muscles. Good night!

Passionflower is surprisingly good for nerve pain and shingles. Shingles are painful. I had a mild case and went to the doctor thinking perhaps my gallbladder was exploding. Helping with the pain and bringing sleep is a gift.

RECOMMENDED DOSAGE: tincture: 25 to 50 drops tincture 3 times a day, but it will make you sleepy—so it's best before bed

CAUTIONS: Not for use in pregnancy or in conjunction with other relaxing or sedating medications. Not for use with MAOIs or blood thinners.

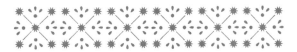

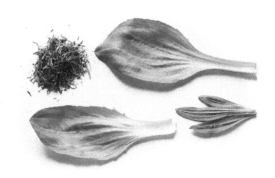

Plantain

LATIN NAME: *Plantago spp.*
ALSO KNOWN NICKNAMES: rabbit ears, ribwort, waybread, waybroad, wagbread, white man's footprint, Englishman's footprint, cuckoo bread, snakeweed, devil's shoestring, common plantain, rabbit ears, ripple grass, healing blade, dooryard plantain, bird seed, rat's tails
FAMILY: Plantaginaceae

A really good reason for getting to know plantain is that it is available to almost everyone. Every time I find myself at an outdoor herb festival, you can be sure you'll see me showing someone to look down beside their shoe, inviting them behind the booth where it's abundant. It came along across the ocean with the colonists and followed them wherever they went. Many seeds came to the colonies, but rarely did they get as far as plantain. It is medicine and food.

QUALITIES: salty, bitter, cool, moist

THERAPEUTIC ACTIONS: alterative, analgesic, anti-inflammatory, anti-microbial, antispasmodic, astringent, decongestant, demulcent, diuretic, drawing, expectorant, refrigerant, tonic, vulnerary

IDEAL FOR ADDRESSING: bladder inflammation, burns, constipation, eczema, gums, hemorrhoids, insect bites, psoriasis, rashes, sore throat, splinters

MEDICINAL PARTS USED: leaves and seeds

COMMON PREPARATIONS: tea, tincture, salve, poultice, soak, oil, vinegar, tub tea, face masks, spit poultices

EFFECTIVE APPLICATIONS: Plantain has drawing properties, which make it great for insect stings and splinters. I found that it worked well at pulling out a salivary gland stone by making tiny poultices of plantain and clay in heat-sealable tea bags. An infusion of plantain is healing and soothing to the digestive system.

RECOMMENDED DOSAGE: considered very safe; tea or tincture: up to 3 times a day, with external use repeated as needed

CAUTIONS: None.

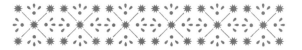

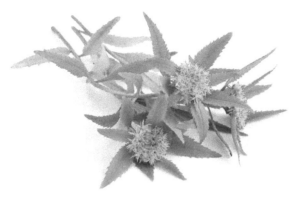

Rhodiola

LATIN NAME: *Rhodiola rosea*
ALSO KNOWN NICKNAMES: golden root, rose root, arctic root
FAMILY: Crassulaceae

Rhodiola is usually sold as small, dried pieces of root that have a soft rose scent, and the flavor of the tincture is agreeably rosy. It grows at high altitudes in mountainous, cold, and rugged regions of Europe, Asia, and parts of North America. There are many pretty wild claims made about this sweet root. That's common with adaptogens, but this one has been approved for various uses in Russia and Sweden, meaning that their research has shown the herb to be capable of improving energy and neurological functions.

QUALITIES: cooling, drying

THERAPEUTIC ACTIONS: adaptogen, antidepressant, antioxidant, cardio-protective, nootropic, stimulant

IDEAL FOR ADDRESSING: anxiety, depression, fatigue, headaches, lack of energy, mental fatigue, inability to concentrate, poor memory, stress, weakness

MEDICINAL PARTS USED: root

COMMON PREPARATIONS: tea, tincture, capsules, tablets

EFFECTIVE APPLICATIONS: Rhodiola is useful for someone who pushes their physical endurance. It drastically reduces recovery time after a workout. As a magazine publisher and writer, I live and die by deadlines. Rhodiola is my best friend when I'm out of time and need to think clearly and focus.

RECOMMENDED DOSAGE: tea: 1 to 2 cups a day; tincture: 20 to 35 drops 1 or 2 times a day. Follow label directions on purchased products.

CAUTIONS: Avoid use if suffering from bipolar disorder. Consult your health care provider before using if pregnant, nursing, or taking medication for emotional issues. Rhodiola is taken on an empty stomach earlier in the day so it doesn't keep you up. It can cause vivid dreams.

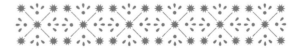

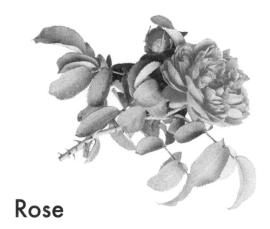

Rose

LATIN NAME: *Rosa spp.*

ALSO KNOWN NICKNAMES: apothecary rose, beach rose, briar hip, briar rose, cabbage rose, damask rose, dogberry, dog rose, eglantine gall, French rose, hep tree, hip fruit, hop fruit, hogseed, multiflora rose, rose hip, sweet briar, witches' briar, wild rose

FAMILY: Rosaceae

Roses are often a gift of love, and it turns out they are a balm to the emotional heart. Oh, they do *so* much more, but that's how most people first think of roses. It comes as a shock to find out that roses are an amazing medicine, capable of taking care of our emotional well-being and a hundred physical issues.

QUALITIES: cooling, moist, sweet

THERAPEUTIC ACTIONS: antidepressant, anti-inflammatory, antiseptic, antispasmodic, antiviral, aphrodisiac, astringent, calming, expectorant, nervine, nourishing, refrigerant, sedative, styptic, tonic

IDEAL FOR ADDRESSING: pain, heat and inflammation from burns (especially sunburn), wounds, scratches, abrasions, rashes, bites, and stings. Trauma, shock, sore throats and mouth sores

MEDICINAL PARTS USED: whole flowers, petals, rosehips

COMMON PREPARATIONS: tea, tincture (glycerite), oil, infused honey, vinegar, flower essence, rosewater, essential oil, soaps, poultices, compresses, lotions

EFFECTIVE APPLICATIONS: My mom's favorite facial preparation was rosewater and glycerin. She found it cooling, soothing, and also firming. The glycerin is a humectant. At the same time, an internal dose or two of rose glycerite for nerves, depression, sadness, and generally being off-kilter is also cooling and soothing and puts you back together.

RECOMMENDED DOSAGE: tea, tincture, or glycerite can safely be used by the dropperful as desired. External use is very gentle and safe.

CAUTIONS: No warnings other than possible allergy. Rose hips have small hairs inside the seed capsule, so avoid piercing or strain well if used for tea.

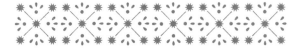

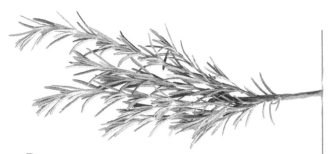

Rosemary

LATIN NAME: *Salvia rosmarinus*, formerly *Rosmarinus officinalis*

ALSO KNOWN NICKNAMES: dew of the sea, old man, compass-weed, compass plant

FAMILY: Lamiaceae

People usually get to know rosemary as a culinary herb, perhaps never considering the medicinal properties it possesses. When a culinary herb is aromatic (as most are), that means that it produces miniscule amounts of essential oils. Aromatic herbs get certain properties from essential oils, and they all strongly promote good health. Sage and thyme will have many of the properties shown with rosemary. Put these bright flavors in your meals.

QUALITIES: warm, dry, pungent, stimulating

THERAPEUTIC ACTIONS: analgesic, antibacterial, anti-fungal, anti-inflammatory, antioxidant, antirheumatic, antiseptic, antispasmodic, antiviral, aromatic, carminative, digestive, diuretic, emmenagogue, mild laxative, nervine, neuroprotective, stimulant, tonic, vulnerary

IDEAL FOR ADDRESSING: anxiety, circulation, concentration, cramping and excess gas, dandruff, mild depression, eczema, exhaustion, stress, weakness

MEDICINAL PARTS USED: stems, leaves, flowers

COMMON PREPARATIONS: tea, tincture, infused oil, vinegar, capsules, often used in cooking

EFFECTIVE APPLICATIONS: Recently there has been a move toward using bar soap as shampoo to reduce packaging waste. That can leave the hair cuticle open, and a vinegar rinse closes it. Try infusing rosemary in vinegar for a couple weeks, strain, and add twice as much water as vinegar. Use a cup or two (depending on hair length) immediately after rinsing out the soap. Rosemary is great for the scalp!

Rosemary tea can revive and energize you without the need for caffeine.

RECOMMENDED DOSAGE: Using rosemary in food is generally a safe quantity, but tea or tincture should be kept to no more than 2 doses daily when needed.

CAUTIONS: Rosemary can also interfere with some medications, such as anticoagulants, blood pressure medications, and diuretics.

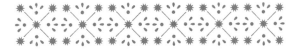

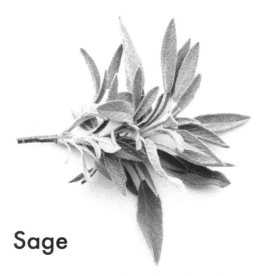

Sage

LATIN NAME: *Salvia officinalis, Salvia spp.*
ALSO KNOWN NICKNAMES: sage, common sage, garden sage, golden sage, kitchen sage, true sage, culinary sage, Dalmatian sage, tri-color sage, purple sage, clary sage, smudge, broadleaf sage
FAMILY: Lamiaceae

Sage is too often thought of as just for use at Thanksgiving. There are so many other reasons to get to know it, and that's not just because it grows into a striking, lush plant that provides usable leaves well into the cold weather season. Sage tea is surprisingly delicious and has a ton of benefits. Many of us know white sage (*Salvia apiana*) as what is often used as a smudge or incense to clear a space of negativity, but any sage at all will work, as will various other native plants. Sage has a stunning array of medicinal properties, too.

QUALITIES: warm, dry, slightly bitter

THERAPEUTIC ACTIONS: alertness and attention span, antibacterial, antifungal, anti-inflammatory, antirheumatic, antiseptic, antispasmodic, astringent, antiviral, carminative

IDEAL FOR ADDRESSING: bad breath and sore gums, spastic cough, depression, poor digestion, joint pain, viral or bacterial infection, upper respiratory infection, dry up milk production, oily skin or hair, mucous membrane wounds, memory loss, sore throat, upset stomach

MEDICINAL PARTS USED: leaf

COMMON PREPARATIONS: tea, vinegar, fresh, tincture, smudge, gargle, mouthwash

EFFECTIVE APPLICATIONS: Sage tea is exceptional for sore throats. It is also useful to help mothers dry up milk if they intend to end nursing.

RECOMMENDED DOSAGE: tea: 3 to 4 cups a day max; tincture: 30 to 60 drops up to 3 times a day

CAUTIONS: Avoid in pregnancy or breast-feeding. Avoid higher amounts for an extended time in pregnancy or during breastfeeding.

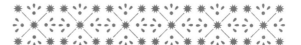

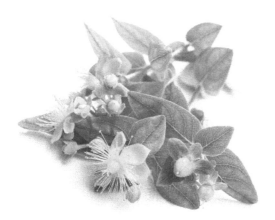

St. John's Wort

LATIN NAME: *Hypericum perforatum*
ALSO KNOWN NICKNAMES: St. Joan's wort
FAMILY: Hypericeae

St. John's wort was a true gateway herb for thousands if not millions of people. In the late 1990s, the TV show *60 Minutes* ran a segment about German research showing St. John's wort's efficacy for depression. Immediately, people who wouldn't have considered herbal medicine became interested. It was the first time that I'm aware of that an herb was scientifically approved.

There are a lot of different varieties of hypericum, and many are used in landscaping. The only one that we use medicinally is the *perforatum*, and to tell it is the right one, hold a leaf up to the light and you'll see tiny pinpricks, or perforations. Alternatively, rub one of the bright yellow flowers between your fingers, and there will be a red dye left behind.

QUALITIES: cooling, slightly bitter, mildly sweet, mild astringent

THERAPEUTIC ACTIONS: analgesic, antidepressant, anti-inflammatory, antiseptic, antiviral, nervine, vulnerary

IDEAL FOR ADDRESSING: anxiety, mild to moderate depression, eczema, insomnia, symptoms of menopause, nerve pain, nervous tension, neuralgia, PMS, restlessness, SAD, viruses, wound healing

MEDICINAL PARTS USED: flowering tops, top 6 inches or so

COMMON PREPARATIONS: tincture, tea, infused oil, pills, capsules

EFFECTIVE APPLICATIONS: Infused olive oil is very good for nerve pain (externally), and it is also very helpful for eczema. Of course the tea, tincture, or capsules can help with depression, too.

RECOMMENDED DOSAGE: tincture: 25 to 50 drops up to 2 or 3 times a day; tea: up to 3 times a day; pills and capsules: follow directions on labels

CAUTIONS: Should not be taken in conjunction with certain medications, especially antidepressant or antianxiety medicines but also contraceptives, blood thinners, antibiotics, and others. Check with your doctor if you're using prescribed medications. May increase sun sensitivity.

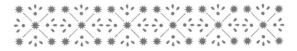

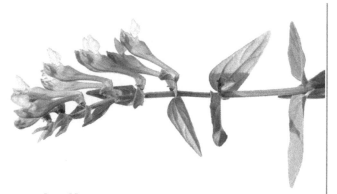

Skullcap

LATIN NAME: *Scutellaria lateriflora*
ALSO KNOWN NICKNAMES: hoodwort, helmet flower, mad dog weed, mad dog skullcap
FAMILY: Lamiaceae

Skullcap has quite a history of use. At one time, because of the sedating property, it was given for rabies (resulting in the "mad dog weed" nickname), and various Native American tribes used it for different things, including aspects of childbirth and recovery, teething pain, and diarrhea, to name just a few. Gradually, it has become known for the way it assists with mood, nerves, spasms, and digestion.

Please use reliable sources (check Resources, page 151). Skullcap has been adulterated with a plant named *germander* in the past.

QUALITIES: cool, dry, relaxing

THERAPEUTIC ACTIONS: antispasmodic, antianxiety, carminative, hypotensive. mood-enhancing, nervine, sedative

IDEAL FOR ADDRESSING: anxiety, nervous headaches, hysteria, indigestion, insomnia, nervousness, muscle cramps, pain, panic attacks, stress

MEDICINAL PARTS USED: aerial parts

COMMON PREPARATIONS: tincture, tea

EFFECTIVE APPLICATIONS: Skullcap is great when you need to relax or get past some nervous tension or anxiety but not pass out so that it's possible to get things done. It's a great remedy for muscle spasms and cramps. A nice cup of tea or some tincture, and very quickly there is relief.

RECOMMENDED DOSAGE: tincture: 40 to 80 drops up to 3 times a day, tea: 3 times a day; capsules: follow directions on manufacturer's label

CAUTIONS: *Do not* use in pregnancy or during breastfeeding. There are varying opinions on whether overuse causes liver damage, so err on the side of caution. Do not overuse; follow directions for use on package or see the preceding notes.

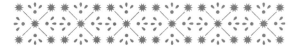

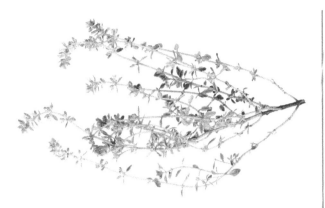

Thyme

LATIN NAME: *Thymus vulgaris*
ALSO KNOWN NICKNAMES: common thyme, garden thyme
FAMILY: Lamiaceae

Thyme is one of the easiest herbs to learn to cook with because it enhances almost any savory dish, from eggs to pasta to beef. Keep a jar of dried thyme (preferably freshly dried from the summer garden) handy so it is easy to toss into dishes as they are prepared. Fresh is even better. First you'll get all the health benefits from the herb, but then it will gradually lead you to try new herbs. All the culinary herbs have terrific health benefits, so let thyme show you the way.

QUALITIES: hot, dry, pungent

THERAPEUTIC ACTIONS: antibiotic, antifungal, antimicrobial, antispasmodic, antiviral, carminative, expectorant, mood enhancing, relaxing

IDEAL FOR ADDRESSING: acute bronchitis, cough, mental fatigue, excess gas, insomnia, sore throat, stress

MEDICINAL PARTS USED: leaves

COMMON PREPARATIONS: tea, tincture, poultice, syrup, vinegar

EFFECTIVE APPLICATIONS: Two tablespoons of thyme in a cup of boiled water is surprisingly tasty and an effective pick-me-up, throat rescue, and mood assist. It's great for coughs, too—just a simple, single-herb tea can do so much.

Thyme tea can also help with a sore throat, indigestion, and coughing and will help bring relaxation.

RECOMMENDED DOSAGE: tincture or tea: up to 3 times a day, culinary use to taste is unlimited (within reason)

CAUTIONS: Avoid in the conditions of epilepsy, pregnancy and high blood pressure.

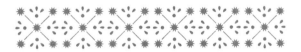

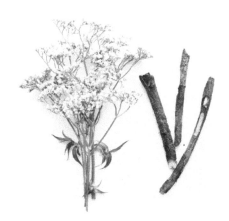

Valerian

LATIN NAME: *Valeriana officinalis*
ALSO KNOWN NICKNAMES: garden heliotrope, common valerian, all-heal
FAMILY: Valerianaceae

Valerian has often been referred to as "herbal valium" because it is relaxing and the names are vaguely similar, but they are in no way related. It's more likely that the pharmaceutical company chose the name because it wanted to be the "chemical valerian." Valerian doesn't have any of the issues that come with benzodiazepines.

QUALITIES: warm, slightly drying

THERAPEUTIC ACTIONS: antispasmodic, anxiolytic, relaxing nervine, sedative

IDEAL FOR ADDRESSING: anxiety, dizziness, hysteria, insomnia, muscle tension, muscular spasms, menstrual cramps and menopause symptoms, nervous tension, and palpitations, spasms

MEDICINAL PARTS USED: roots, leaves, flowers

COMMON PREPARATIONS: powder, tea, tincture, capsules

EFFECTIVE APPLICATIONS: Valerian most often comes to mind for trouble sleeping. Capsules or tincture are preferred because of the scent of valerian. Some people (me, for instance) have the opposite reaction to valerian, so try it sometime during the day rather than worsening insomnia.

If you can find tincture or tea made with valerian flowers, they have a gentler action, and I like them because they relax me rather than jazzing me up like the roots. Also, the fresh flowers smell so incredibly beautiful that after you've smelled them you recognize that scent in the roots and can drink tea made from roots more easily. Valerian is very easy to grow, and that's a good way to get the flowers.

RECOMMENDED DOSAGE: tea: up to 3 times a day for anxiety; for sleep, 2 capsules or 40 drops up to an hour before bedtime

CAUTIONS: Should not be taken with alcohol or medications for depression or sleep.

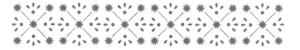

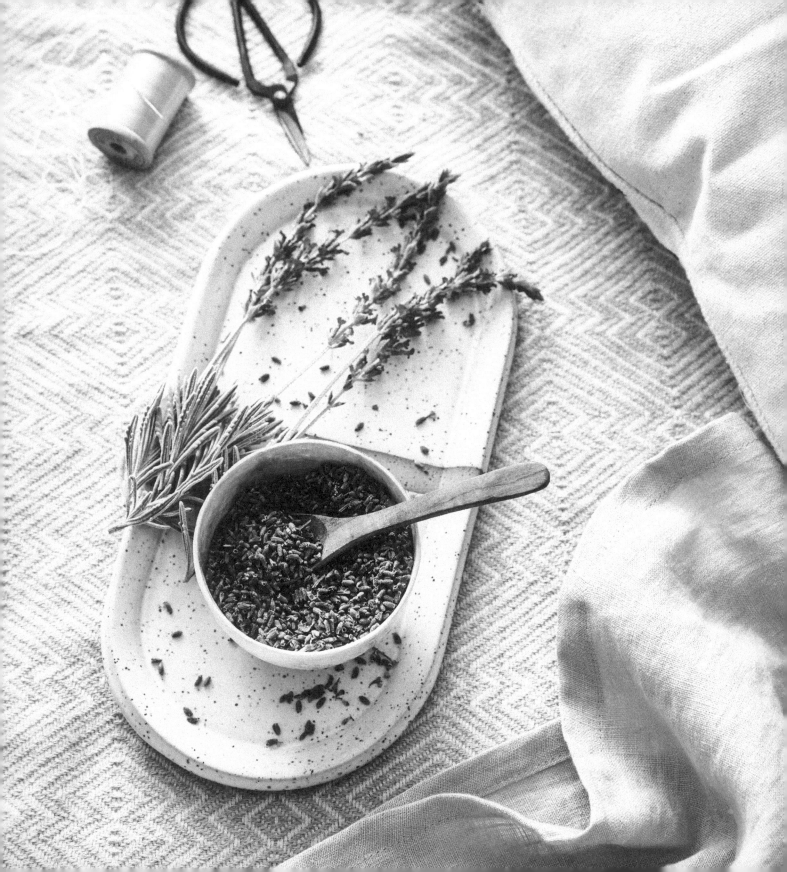

Glossary

ADAPTOGEN – A class of nontoxic herbs that balance, restore, and protect the body

ADRENAL TONIC – A tonic that supports, tones, and nourishes adrenal glands

ALTERATIVE – Cures or restores health by changing processes in the body

ANALGESIC – A substance that reduces or eliminates pain while one stays awake

ANODYNE – Synonymous with analgesic

ANTIBACTERIAL – Inhibits growth of or kills bacteria

ANTIBIOTIC – Destroys or inhibits growth of microorganisms

ANTIDEPRESSANT – Substance that lessens depression

ANTIDIABETIC – Helps control blood glucose levels

ANTIFUNGAL – Inhibits fungal growth or kills fungus

ANTIHISTAMINE – Blocks histamine reaction

ANTI-INFLAMMATORY – Reduces the body's immune response to injury, infection, or irritant

ANTIOXIDANT – Protects cells against the effects of free radicals

ANTISEPTIC – Prevents infection from microorganisms

ANTISPASMODIC – Relieves or relaxes spasms

ANTITUSSIVE – Suppresses cough

ANTIVIRAL – Inhibits or kills viruses

ANXIOLYTIC – Reduces anxiety

APHRODISIAC – Increases and/or improves intimacy and sexual desire

ASTRINGENT – Shrinks or constricts tissue

CARMINATIVE – Encourages the release of gas from stomach and intestines

DECOCTION – A "tea" of bark, root, or seeds that requires boiling or simmering in water

DECONGESTANT – Relieves congestion in the upper respiratory system

DEMULCENT – Substance that produces a soothing coating over mucus membranes

DIURETIC – Stimulates the elimination of urine

EMOLLIENT – Soothing to skin or mucus membrane

EXPECTORANT – Promotes the expulsion of mucus from air passages

GALACTAGOGUE – Increases the secretion of milk

HEPATIC – Refers to the liver

HYPNOTIC – Induces sleep

IMMUNE TONIC – Supports and tones the immune system

INFUSED OIL – A vegetable oil in which herbs have macerated to release their properties

LAXATIVE – Encourages the production of bowel movements

LYMPHATIC – Deep cleans and improves flow of lymph through the body

MENSTRUUM – Solvent (alcohol, glycerin, vinegar) in which herbs release their properties for tinctures

MUCILAGINOUS – Having a slick, slippery texture

NERVINE – Benefits and supports the nervous system

NEUROPROTECTIVE – Protects neurons from injury or degeneration and protects brain function

NOOTROPIC – Enhances cognitive function, memory, and learning

PECTORAL – Tones and strengthens the pulmonary system

PULSING – To take a substance for a period of time, take a short break, and resume

PURGATIVE – Strong laxative

RELAXANT – Calms without sedating; relaxes contracted tissues

SEDATIVE – Calms or moderates nervousness and excitement

STIMULANT – Creates movement and/or energy

STYPTIC – Stops bleeding, usually on contact

TONIC – Restore or increase body or tissue tone

VASODILATOR – Opens blood vessels by relaxing muscular vessel walls

VULNERARY – Helps wounds heal

Herbal Ally Substitutes

The herbs chosen for this book are all pretty easy and safe to work with, but of course, they do need to be treated with respect. Ideally before beginning to make substitutions, you can get to know them one at a time and pay attention to how your body reacts to them.

If any herbs are new to you or if working with a particular formulation is new, work with simple combinations. Unless the symptom or condition has very clear energetic qualities (dry/moist, hot/cold, etc.), try to balance the formula by choosing herbs that energetically work together. For instance, a drying herb might benefit from the addition of a moistening herb like plantain or marshmallow. A cooling herb could use some ginger, which is warming.

We tried to choose herbs that were readily available, but it isn't always possible to get the exact herbal ingredient listed in the remedies section. Should you need to make a substitution, check the therapeutic actions of that herb and select an herb that has several of the same actions. As you become more comfortable working with herbs, you may find this chart helpful for creating your own recipes.

Lastly, start with a low dose of a new blend, and work up *only if necessary*.

ADAPTOGENS
ashwagandha
astragalus
eleuthero
holy basil
rhodiola

ALTERATIVE
ashwagandha
elder
plantain

ANALGESIC
blue vervain
California poppy
echinacea
ginger
ginkgo
holy basil
mimosa
nettle
plantain
rose
rosemary
St. John's wort

ANTIBACTERIAL
astragalus
chamomile
echinacea
ginger
holy basil
mint
motherwort
nettle
plantain
rose
sage
thyme

ANTIBIOTIC
catnip
lavender
thyme

ANTICOAGULANT
ginger

ANTIDEPRESSANT
holy basil
lavender
lemon balm
oat

ANTIDEPRESSANT

(continued)

passionflower

rhodiola

rose

St. John's wort

ANTIDIABETIC

eleuthero

ANTIFUNGAL

echinacea

ginger

holy basil

lavender

mint

motherwort

rosemary

sage

thyme

ANTIHISTAMINE

chamomile

mint

nettle

ANTI-HYPERTENSIVE

hawthorn

ANTI-INFLAMMATORY

ashwagandha

astragalus

chamomile

echinacea

elder

ginger

ginkgo

hawthorn

holy basil

lavender

marshmallow

mint

nettle

plantain

rose

rosemary

sage

St. John's wort

ANTIOXIDANT

echinacea

elder

hawthorn

holy basil

lemon balm

mint

motherwort

rhodiola

rosemary

ANTISEPTIC

ashwagandha

echinacea

lavender

rose

rosemary

sage

St. John's wort

ANTISPASMODIC

ashwagandha

blue vervain

California poppy

catnip

lavender

lemon balm

marshmallow

motherwort

passionflower

plantain

rose

rosemary

sage

skullcap

thyme

valerian

ANTITUSSIVE

ashwagandha

marshmallow

ANTIVIRAL

astragalus

echinacea

elder

eleuthero

ginger

holy basil

lavender

lemon balm

rose

rosemary

sage

St. John's wort

thyme

ANXIOLYTIC

ashwagandha

California poppy

ginkgo

hawthorn

holy basil

mint

passionflower

skullcap

valerian

APHRODISIAC

ashwagandha

rose

ASTRINGENT

echinacea

elder

hawthorn

motherwort

nettle

plantain

rose

sage

BITTER

blue vervain

chamomile

CARDIOTONIC

hawthorn

motherwort

CARDIO-PROTECTANT

rhodiola

CARMINATIVE

chamomile
ginger
hawthorn
lavender
lemon balm
mimosa
mint
rosemary
sage
skullcap
thyme

CIRCULATORY STIMULANT

ginkgo
hawthorn
motherwort

DECONGESTANT

nettle
plantain

DEMULCENT

elder
marshmallow
plantain

DIAPHORETIC

catnip
ginger
motherwort

DIURETIC

astragalus
blue vervain
elder
ginkgo
hawthorn
holy basil
marshmallow
mimosa
motherwort
nettle
plantain
rosemary

EMMENAGOGUE

motherwort
rosemary

EXPECTORANT

blue vervain
elder
holy basil
nettle
plantain
rose
thyme

GALACTAGOGUE

catnip

HEPATIC

lavender

HYPOTENSIVE

passionflower
skullcap

HYPNOTIC

California poppy
passionflower

IMMUNE SYSTEM SUPPORT

ashwagandha
astragalus
catnip
echinacea
elder
ginger
holy basil
motherwort

LAXATIVE

elder
motherwort
rosemary

MOOD-ENHANCING

mimosa
skullcap
thyme

NERVINE

blue vervain
California poppy
catnip
holy basil
lemon balm
mimosa
motherwort
oat
passionflower
rose

rosemary
skullcap
St. John's wort
valerian

NEURO-PROTECTIVE

eleuthero
ginger
holy basil
rosemary

NOOTROPIC

ashwagandha
ginkgo
lemon balm
rhodiola

NUTRITIVE

nettle
oats
rose

REFRIGERANT

mint
plantain
rose

RELAXANT

blue vervain
catnip
hawthorn
lavender
mimosa
thyme
valerian

SEDATIVE

ashwagandha

blue vervain

California poppy

catnip

chamomile

lavender

lemon balm

mimosa

motherwort

rose

skullcap

valerian

STIMULANT

ashwagandha

mimosa

rhodiola

rosemary

STYPTIC

nettle

rose

THERMOGENIC

ginger

TONIC

astragalus

echinacea

eleuthero

holy basil

marshmallow

mimosa

motherwort

nettle

plantain

rose

rosemary

VASODILATOR

astragalus

motherwort

VULNERARY

echinacea

marshmallow

mimosa

plantain

rosemary

St. John's wort

Measurement Conversions

Simpler's Method of Measurement

For this book, I used specific measurements, but in my own recipe books I measure in parts, called the simpler's method. Using this method, the specific unit of measurement is not important; it's about the proportion. Usually "parts" refers to measurement by volume—not weight. Here's an example:

THIS TEA BLEND IN PARTS:

2 parts chamomile

1 part spearmint

COULD BE INTERPRETED AS:

2 tablespoons chamomile

1 tablespoon spearmint

OR

2 cups chamomile

1 cup spearmint

OR

2 barrels chamomile

1 barrel spearmint

WEIGHT EQUIVALENTS

US Standard	Metric (approximate)
½ ounce	15 g
1 ounce	30 g
2 ounces	60 g
4 ounces	115 g
8 ounces	225 g
12 ounces	340 g
16 ounces or 1 pound	455 g

VOLUME EQUIVALENTS (LIQUID)

US Standard	US Standard (ounces)	Metric (approximate)
2 tablespoons	1 fl. oz.	30 mL
¼ cup	2 fl. oz.	60 mL
½ cup	4 fl. oz.	120 mL
1 cup	8 fl. oz.	240 mL
1½ cups	12 fl. oz.	355 mL
2 cups or 1 pint	16 fl. oz.	475 mL
4 cups or 1 quart	32 fl. oz.	1 L
1 gallon	128 fl. oz.	4 L

VOLUME EQUIVALENTS (DRY)

US Standard	Metric (approximate)
⅛ teaspoon	0.5 mL
¼ teaspoon	1 mL
½ teaspoon	2 mL
¾ teaspoon	4 mL
1 teaspoon	5 mL
1 tablespoon	15 mL
¼ cup	59 mL
⅓ cup	79 mL
½ cup	118 mL
⅔ cup	156 mL
¾ cup	177 mL
1 cup	235 mL
2 cups or 1 pint	475 mL
3 cups	700 mL
4 cups or 1 quart	1 L

OVEN TEMPERATURES

Fahrenheit (F)	Celsius (C) (approximate)
250°F	120°C
300°F	150°C
325°F	165°C
350°F	180°C
375°F	190°C
400°F	200°C
425°F	220°C
450°F	230°C

Resources

I'm not much of a seed starter, and it so happens that in my part of the world there are lots of wonderful herb festivals each spring. We also have many small, family-run herb farms in the county. It's easy for me to find herbal plant starters. Many small farmers don't sell online because they're out weeding and pinching and watering, but they're worth finding. Shop local whenever you can.

Seeds

All of these provide non-GMO, heirloom, quality seeds.
SouthernExposure.com
JohnnySeeds.com
RareSeeds.com

Seeds and Plants

I just picked up some eleuthero seeds from Strictly Medicinal. Just about any medicinal plant/seed you're looking for can be found here. Great selection, prices, and service.
StrictlyMedicinalSeeds.com

Herbs and Supplies

I tried to choose suppliers from different parts of the United States, keeping shipping in mind. As mentioned previously, shop locally if possible. We want those local apothecaries to do well and stay open!

Dandelion Botanicals, Seattle, Washington
DandelionBotanical.com
Sells by the ounce (weight) and very reasonable. Family owned. Tons of preparations.

Flower Essence Society, FES, Nevada City, California
FESFlowers.com
Reputable source for high-quality flower essences, many created from their bio-dynamic farm.

Penn Herb, Philadelphia, Pennsylvania
PennHerb.com
Very well established with all kinds of herbs and preparations.

Red Moon Herbs, Asheville, North Carolina
RedMoonHerbs.com
Limited bulk herbs, but a beautiful line of herbal products.

Voyage Botanica, New Mexico

VoyageBotanica.net

Hand-gathered and processed from the Southwest. Seasonally available fresh local roots and herbs.

Blessed Maine Herbs, Athens, Maine

BlessedMaineHerbs.com

Beautiful tinctures, elixirs, balms, syrups, and more. Seasonally available herbs grown on their farm.

The Rosemary House, Mechanicsburg, Pennsylvania

www.therosemaryhouse.com

Lots of dried herbs and tinctures of all sorts.

Mountain Rose Herbs, Eugene, Oregon

MountainRoseHerbs.com

Everything!

Bottles and Jars

Both sources have an amazing selection of bottles, jars, tins, vials, lip balm containers, and more. Glass is heavy to ship, so I've listed locations so you can choose the closest.

New York and Nevada: SKS Bottle & Packaging

SKS-Bottle.com

Seattle and Nashville: Specialty Bottle

SpecialtyBottle.com

Learn More

The Essential Herbal Magazine

EssentialHerbal.com

Down-to-earth and focused on all areas of herbalism for everyone from beginners to experts.

Herb Mentor

LearningHerbs.com

A monthly subscription that supplies a forum with video, articles, and all kinds of information.

There are currently more online herb schools than I can list here. The best thing to do is join one of the many Facebook groups about herbs and ask for opinions. They are all slightly different, and you can ask specific questions. My group is Facebook.com/groups/theessentialherbal.

Get Help

National Suicide Prevention Lifeline
1-800-273-8255
SuicidePreventionLifeline.org
If you have thoughts of harming yourself or are experiencing emotional distress, you can get free and confidential help by calling the suicide prevention lifeline. You can also chat with someone online at the organizationmotwebsite, too.

References

Glausiusz, Josie. "Is Dirt the New Prozac?" *Discover Magazine* (July 13, 2007). Accessed March 4, 2020. DiscoverMagazine.com/mind/is-dirt-the-new -prozac.

Scudellari, Megan. "Your Body Is Teeming with Weed Receptors." *The Scientist* (July 16, 2017). Accessed March 4, 2020. The-Scientist. com/features/your-body-is-teeming-with-wee d-receptors-31233.

Walker, Cathy. "The Beauty of Making Your Own Medicine." *The Essential Herbal* (January/February 2020): 18.

Index

Acknowledgments

In PA and beyond, we were so deeply blessed to have had the glorious Bertha Reppert nearby at her shop The Rosemary House in Mechanicsburg. She blazed a trail here, and I believe she is responsible for our rich and generous herbal scene that continues to grow, evolve, and welcome new herbies.

Although the old-timers had indigenous plant knowledge blended with Pennsylvania German (Amish, etc.) herb use, it had become buried under modern medicine. In fact, even culinary herb use was rare. Her vast writings and endless teaching changed that. Her daughters Susanna and Nancy have continued the tradition she started.

In each area, there is someone who sets the tone, and if you're really lucky, it is someone like Bertha Reppert. She taught all of us to want to spread around the love of herbs. Here's to you, Mrs. Reppert. Thank you.

About the Author

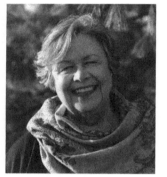

TINA SAMS has loved learning about plants from the time she was a small child but didn't get to chuck her corporate job and play in the dirt until her early 30s. She and her sister stumbled into owning an herb shop at a renaissance festival, and everything bloomed from there. Learning how to take care of her family first drew her in, but eventually foraging wild herbs for food and medicine took over.

In 2002, she started publishing *The Essential Herbal* magazine, and she has a ball doing it.

It's a perfect excuse to plant her so-called yard with herbs, edible plants, medicinal and fruit trees, and even some plants she hasn't had time to get to know yet.

She's written several books and has no intention of slowing down.